GERIATRIC
PEARLS

GERIATRIC PEARLS

MOIRA FORDYCE, MD, FRCP Ed

Clinical Associate Professor
University of California, San Francisco
San Francisco, California
Clinical Professor
Stanford University School of Medicine
Stanford, California

F. A. DAVIS COMPANY • Philadelphia

F. A. Davis Company
1915 Arch Street
Philadelphia, PA 19103

Printed in Canada
Last digit indicates print number: 10 9 8 7 6 5 4 3 2

Medical Publisher: Robert W. Reinhardt
Senior Developmental Editor: Bernice M. Wissler
Production Editor: Jessica Howie Martin
Cover Designer: Louis J. Forgione

As new scientific information becomes available through basic and clinical research, recommended treatments and drug therapies undergo changes. The author and publisher have done everything possible to make this book accurate, up to date, and in accord with accepted standards at the time of publication. The author, editors, and publisher are not responsible for errors or omissions or for consequences from application of the book, and make no warranty, expressed or implied, in regard to the contents of the book. Any practice described in this book should be applied by the reader in accordance with professional standards of care used in regard to the unique circumstances that may apply in each situation. The reader is advised always to check product information (package inserts) for changes and new information regarding dose and contraindications before administering any drug. Caution is especially urged when using new or infrequently ordered drugs.

Library of Congress Cataloging-in-Publication Data
Fordyce, Moira. 1939–
   Geriatric pearls/Moira Fordyce.
   p. cm.
   Includes bibliographical references and index.
   ISBN 0-8036-0434-3 (alk. paper)
   1. Geriatrics Handbooks, manuals, etc. I. Title.
   [DNLM: 1. Geriatrics Handbooks. 2. Aging—physiology Handbooks.
3. Geriatric Assessment Handbooks. 4. Drug Therapy—Aged Handbooks.
5. Terminal Care—Aged Handbooks. WT 39 F713g 1999]
RC952.55.F67 1999
618.97—dc21
DNLM/DLC
For Library of Congress   99-13819
                                                                CIP

Preface

"Dr. Fordyce, we're overwhelmed! We can't face another big textbook, but we all know how important geriatrics is and will continue to be. Can you help us?" This cry from the hearts of the family practice residents whom I was teaching led me to write this book. In draft form, it was enthusiastically received by nurses; nurse practitioners; physician assistants; medical social workers; medical students; and doctors, both in training and well established. A number of the latter told me that it had proved a great aid for quick review of the subject. Interest in the book has also been expressed by chiropractors and physical therapists. Nursing home directors and staff members have asked me when they can have a copy.

There are several reasons for this intense interest. First is the aging of the population. By the year 2010, which is not far away, 1 out of 5 Americans will be 65 or older, with all the accompanying health and functional problems. Almost all health professionals will have some contact with the elderly in their professional or personal life or both. The second reason for this interest is the manageable size of the book, which, although small, is full of useful information. Its practical advice, mnemonics, and many tables make it an ideal, quick reference to carry in a pocket. The third reason for this interest is that, despite the large number of elderly patients in acute and chronic care facilities, the teaching of geriatrics is still neglected in most medical and nursing schools.

The topics covered in *Geriatric Pearls* include changes with normal aging (How can disease be recognized without clear understanding of what's normal?); geriatric evaluation and its importance; common geriatric syndromes, diseases, and injuries; and a detailed look at managing medications in the elderly. The value of rehabilitation in different settings is presented, and the book concludes with practical and philosophical advice on end-of-life issues, another important but sadly neglected topic.

Currently, great emphasis is placed on the *science* of medicine—the seductive lure of high-tech investigations and procedures. Unfortunately, for many health professionals the *art* of medicine has become undervalued and sometimes lost completely. Patients are aware of this difference and, although wishing for the best that modern medicine has to offer, are drawn to the practitioner who listens to them, looks at them, and touches them. They want the practitioner to be able to combine the best of both worlds—high tech (but with good judgment about futile treatments) and caring. The importance of this art of medicine, which has survived through the centuries, tested and true, pervades this book. I hope that this aspect of the book will provide a quiet center in our whirlwind medical world for the health professionals who use it.

MOIRA FORDYCE
SAN FRANCISCO

Acknowledgments

I wish to thank the following people for their help, patience, and ongoing support throughout the writing of this book:

My husband Alastair and my sons Alexander, Niall, and Graeme. All four are a constant source of love and inspiration for me.

Significant others who have helped and encouraged me are Diane N. Christenson, PA-C; Lucinda Hirahoka-Pisano, PA-C; William C. Fowkes, MD; Donald Bardole, MD; Owen M. Lum, MD; and Robert M. Norman, MD.

My thanks to the American Geriatrics Society for encouraging me to include their guidelines, "Current Guidelines for Practice: Oral Anticoagulation for Older Adults."

Last, but by no means least, I want to thank my excellent editor, Bernice M. Wissler, for her patience and skill.

A Note about Terminology

To achieve economy of words, this text often uses the terms "the elderly," "elders," or "seniors" to refer to older people in general. Their meaning is not intended to be negative in any way.

Contents

APPENDIXES

PART

Normal Aging

*The first forty years of life give us the text; the
next thirty supply the commentary.*
Arthur Schopenhauer (1788–1860)

1
CHAPTER

Physiological Changes with Aging

Senescence begins
And middle age ends
The day your descendants
Outnumber your friends.
Ogden Nash (1902–1971), *Crossing the Border*

Everything in the physical world eventually wears out. Our bodies deteriorate with living. There is no potion, spell, or bargain we can make with god or demon that can change this. No one escapes. As you read this, *you* are growing older. Aging is living—keep living long enough and you will find that you are old. Aging brings all living things closer to death. The death of an elderly person, although sad, is neither a triumph nor a defeat. It is inevitable and is the normal end of life.

Fortunately, the mind, the spirit, and creativity need not deteriorate. On the contrary, they can continue to grow as long as we are alive.

The elderly are more fragile than the young. Displacement from homeostasis occurs more easily, reserve in body systems decreases, and recovery from disease or injury is slower and often incomplete. All the body systems, including the immune system, function less efficiently. Aches and pains accumulate. Drugs of all kinds—prescription, over-the-counter, alternative medicines, alcohol, caffeine—have a more powerful effect on body and mind.

VARIABILITY

Variability Within the Group

The longer people live, the less like anyone else they become—the members of a group at age 70 are less similar to each other than they were at age 30—physically, mentally, and spiritually. We should remember too that the long-lived, even if they seem frail, are the tough ones, the survivors; we should be proud of them and value their memories and life experience.

Variability Within the Individual

Variability can also be seen within each individual because body systems do not necessarily age at the same rate. Because each patient increasingly becomes one of a kind with the passage of time, diagnosis and treatment of disease in the elderly are a challenge. Women tend to live longer than men, but often in poorer health.

STARTING POINT

The point from which a human being starts is significant. At any age, a highly trained athlete can become less fit and still be above average. The lively mind, interested in everything and willing to be involved, keeps new cellular connections growing in the brain throughout life.

People usually become more like what they already are in personality as they age: the mellow become even more so and the "crabby" and difficult even worse. The fearful panic more easily, and the kind and generous are wonderful to have around. I have looked after some nasty elders, but no dull ones. Optimists generally age more successfully than do pessimists.

RIGIDITY

Rigidity of body or mind at any age acts against optimal function and satisfaction with life.

CHANGES IN BODY AND MIND WITH NORMAL AGING

Eyes

The lens of the eye becomes less elastic, which makes focusing on close objects difficult for the normal or farsighted individual. (This is called presbyopia.) Eyeglasses or contact lenses can compensate for this. Yellow pigment accumulates in the lens and can alter color perception. The iris becomes more rigid, so less light enters the eye. The visual field can shrink, causing "tunneling" of vision. The aging eye is more sensitive to glare at all times, but especially at night. These changes in vision can make driving an automobile more hazardous, especially after dark (because of oncoming headlights) and in heavy traffic. I advise my elderly patients to avoid driving under these conditions.

Dry eyes are common with aging. Artificial tears, preferably without preservatives, help alleviate this condition.

Ears

Loss of high tones occurs, with decreased ability to screen out surrounding noise and focus on individual sounds (presbycusis). Wax in the ears is common and can dull hearing, but is easily removed once it is diagnosed. Deafness, which occurs more often in men, can be mistaken for dementia.

Skin

The skin becomes thinner, dryer, and less elastic. It tears and bruises easily. Dryness can cause troublesome itching. Elderly people should avoid temperature extremes when bathing, and pat (not rub) the skin dry. A vegetable shortening such as Crisco applied on slightly moist skin is a good, inexpensive remedy for dryness. More recommendations for skin care appear in Chapter 2.

Hair and Nails

Hair changes in texture and color. Nails change in texture. These changes don't matter except cosmetically.

Musculoskeletal System

Lean body mass decreases and skeletal muscle fibers are replaced with fatty tissue as we age. Loss of muscle results in decreased strength and endurance, but many studies now show that regular exercise can modify this loss and maintain significant muscle strength at any age. Increase in fatty tissue can permit a buildup of fat-soluble drugs and chemicals in the aging body.

The spine loses length, mainly as a result of thinning of the intervertebral discs and decrease in the intervertebral disc space. Exercise and good posture can positively counteract this change.

Joint cartilage erodes from wear and tear, elastic synovial tissue is replaced by more rigid collagen fibers, and synovial fluid becomes more viscous. These changes lead to a decrease in joint mobility. Exercise such as yoga, which emphasizes flexibility, can counteract these changes.

Total bone mass decreases and bones become more fragile with aging, so trivial injury can produce fracture and loss of function. (See section on "Instability,

Gait Disorders, and Falls" in Chap. 8.) Good diet, no smoking, and regular exercise will keep bones strong with no bad side effects.

Heart

The heart is usually fine at rest and with mild exercise, but with age it becomes less efficient in response to increased demands. Regular exercise can counteract this effect to some extent.

Lungs

The lungs become stiffer and the chest wall becomes less resilient.

Gastrointestinal Tract

Altered motility can occur, with some incoordination of peristalsis. The gut can become more sluggish overall. A diet that is low in fiber and fluid, combined with a lack of exercise, can lead to constipation (see Chap. 8).

Genitourinary System

In women, all tissues become more lax. This laxness can contribute to stress incontinence (see Chap. 8). Vaginal dryness can make sexual intercourse painful (dyspareunia). Estrogen replacement therapy and a lubricant such as K-Y jelly can improve this situation.

In men, the prostate enlarges and can produce difficulty with urination. Normal aging does not cause impotence. If impotence occurs, look for a reason.

As discussed in Chapter 8, normal aging does not cause urinary incontinence.

Sexuality

Men can take longer to achieve full erection and longer to recover after orgasm if a second erection is desired. Medication-induced impotence is a common problem. The precursors to, and production of, female orgasm change relatively little throughout life.

Sexual desire and attitudes toward sex alter very little throughout life. The senior who has enjoyed sex when younger will continue to enjoy it as long as he or she has a partner. The whole spectrum of sexuality and sensuality can be explored and enjoyed at any age.

Nervous System

Reaction time slows with aging. This can make accidents more likely while driving or operating machinery. Balance and coordination can also be impaired, increasing the risk of falling.

Sleep

Quantity

The total amount of sleep needed in 24 hours for the person to feel rested probably stays constant throughout life. It can be divided between afternoon naps and nighttime sleep. Sleeping during the day, however, will mean a shorter time asleep at night.

Quality

The quality of sleep changes with age. There is a longer latent period before falling asleep, there are more frequent awakenings, and sleep is lighter overall. Sedatives are not the answer. They should be prescribed in small amounts for a limited time, for instance, to a grieving person who cannot sleep after the death of a loved one. Even in this case, better long-term solutions would be support from family, friends, and community; counseling; and more exercise. Alcohol is not a good remedy for insomnia because it disrupts normal sleep patterns. Daily exercise improves the quality of sleep.

Waking earlier in the morning and going to sleep earlier at night becomes the pattern for many seniors. This pattern can be countered by a few hours of exposure to bright light in the late afternoon or evening.

Memory

Retrieval of information is slower. New skills can be learned throughout life, but for elders learning might take longer and require more concentration, less interference (quiet versus noisy surroundings), better lighting, and so forth.

Creativity

Living long probably enhances creativity. There are many outstanding examples of elderly genius in every field—art, music, literature. Studies now available confirm that playing a musical instrument feeds the brain at any age. Making music with other people feeds the brain and spirit, as well as the interactive, social side. Writing down personal life experiences stimulates the memory.

THE IMPORTANCE OF FUNCTION

A major difference between being old and being young is that disease, injury, poor nutrition, and adverse social circumstances can have greater effects on basic daily functioning in the elderly. Inability for self-care causes general deterioration, which causes further decrease in function. If this deterioration leads to loss of independence, depression and decreased motivation can result. The consequence of this downward spiral can be a poorer quality of life, followed by an earlier-than-necessary death.

PEARL: The health care provider who focuses on disease in the elderly, to the exclusion of function, contributes to the decline of his or her patients.

Functional assessment is an important part of geriatric evaluation in every setting—acute hospital, medical office, skilled nursing facility, and at home. It is more important to know whether an elderly person can get up from a chair and walk than to record in detail the range of motion of the knee. Knowledge of the patient's baseline level of function before illness is essential for realistic rehabilitation afterwards. (Evaluation and recovery of function are discussed further in Chaps. 4, 7, and 14.)

THE IMPORTANCE OF STAYING MOBILE

Bed rest of more than a day or so causes rapid deconditioning and loss of function at any age, but is more harmful in the elderly. Muscles quickly waste away and appetite decreases. There can be costly physical consequences such as constipation, deep vein thrombosis, pulmonary embolism, development of pressure sores, hypostatic pneumonia, and limb contractures. Mental sequelae can include delirium, depression, and loss of confidence.

PEARL: Encourage your patients of any age to make any period of bed rest brief. Mobilization and rehabilitation should start as early as possible in any illness, and regular exercise should be a part of the daily routine.

2
CHAPTER

Prevention of Disease and Injury

There is no cure for birth and death save to enjoy the interval.
George Santayana (1863–1952)

Adopting a healthy lifestyle can prevent much disease and injury. In this chapter are recommendations aimed at the special needs of the elderly, often expressed as direct advice for the sake of brevity. Figure 2–1 illustrates how many of these recommendations can interact to help an individual age successfully. Chapter 3 explains how you can assess the health and lifestyle of elderly individuals and help them to optimize their health and function and to minimize lifestyle risks.

SENSIBLE NUTRITION

PEARL: The older the patient, the more liberal the diet should be. Nevertheless, certain principles of sensible nutrition should be suggested to most healthy elderly individuals:

- Keep intake of saturated fat low.
- Keep fiber intake high.

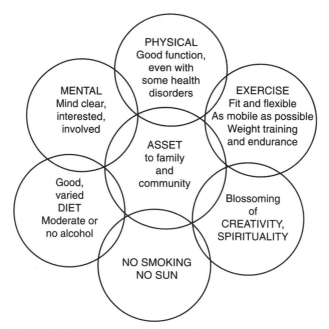

Figure 2–1. Components of successful aging.

- Go easy on salt and sugar.
- An egg is an excellent nutritional package.
- Four ounces of meat or fish daily provides all essential amino acids and many minerals and vitamins.
- Eat fruit and vegetables (lightly cooked or raw) daily.
- Drink enough fluid: a glass of water with each meal and one glass between meals.
- Eat a well-balanced diet. Avoid fad diets; they do not work and can cause damage.
- Enjoyment of food aids digestion and is important at any age.

The healthiest weight range for seniors is **ideal body weight** (IBW) plus up to 10%. A quick, easy formula for calculating IBW follows:

- Measure adult height.

- Women: Allow 100 lb for 5 feet, plus 5 lb for every inch over 5 feet.
- Men: Allow 106 lb for 5 feet, plus 6 lb for every inch over 5 feet.

EXERCISE

Thirty minutes of exercise three times per week is the minimum amount necessary to maintain adequate skeletal muscle mass and tone and to confer benefits on heart, lungs, bones, and mood. Thirty minutes per day is better. Low-impact pursuits such as walking, bicycling, or swimming are kinder to aging joints than high-impact ones such as jogging. Gentle daily exercise such as gardening also confers significant benefit, particularly in very old and frail persons.

A good regimen at any age is a combination of aerobic exercise (such as a brisk walk) for at least 10 minutes, exercising with weights for 10 minutes more, and focusing on flexibility for at least 10 minutes. Yoga and tai chi are both excellent for flexibility, and there are many classes available. Such a daily program is not difficult and has sufficient variety in it to keep up interest. The time can be increased as strength and endurance are built up.

Exercising with friends compounds the benefits and may make it easier to fulfill a regular exercise commitment.

DENTAL CARE

Twice yearly visits to a dentist for cleaning and repair are essential. Recent studies suggest an association between bacteria in plaque and heart disease.

At any age, daily cleaning and flossing of teeth help to fight tooth and gum disease.

SPECIAL SENSES

Healthy elders should have an eye examination every 1 to 2 years and more often if a disease such as diabetes is present. Hearing should be tested as needed.

SKIN CARE

To protect the skin, not just the elderly, but people of all ages should:

- Avoid direct sun, tanning salons, and very hot or cold water.
- Apply sunscreen with sun protection factor (SPF) 15 or more, 30 minutes before every sun exposure. Reapply often.
- Wear a shady hat or carry a parasol. Stay out of the midday sun.
- Avoid soap if the skin is dry or sensitive. Keri lotion or oil (or the generic equivalent) is a good, nondrying body cleanser.
- Learn skin and mucosal self-inspection and do it every week.

SUBSTANCE USE

Advise elderly people:

- **PEARL: Do not use tobacco.**
- Use alcohol moderately or not at all.

SAFETY

More accidents occur at home than anywhere else, so common sense dictates that it's worth giving thought to safety at home as well as in the car. Some injury-prevention advice is valid for all ages, and some principles apply especially to seniors.

Home

A full-scale home safety evaluation is usually done only when a patient is coming home from the hospital or from a skilled nursing facility, but it makes good sense for everyone to take similar precautions. It is not difficult to evaluate home conditions and incorporate the kind of safety equipment and precautions listed in Chapter 14.

Automobile

Elderly drivers have more accidents and injuries per mile driven than do younger adults. Safety principles such as those that follow can minimize accidents and injuries:

- Use seat belts.
- Avoid night driving.
- Avoid heavy traffic.
- Be sure that it is safe for you to drive. Ask your doctor about the effects of medications.
- Do not use alcohol.
- Take the 8-hour training course, "55 Alive," offered by the American Association of Retired Persons (AARP). (Besides safety, another benefit is an auto insurance discount.)
- Have vision checked yearly.

AARP, HMOs, and hospitals have safety self-assessment check lists and videos, some free to borrow, some to buy. In some states, an advanced driving test is offered. Many insurance companies give a 10% discount on auto insurance to those who pass.

HORMONE REPLACEMENT THERAPY

The use of estrogen in postmenopausal women (even those over 70, if they have no contraindications) can have considerable benefits, including decreased osteoporosis; favorable cardiovascular effects (lower incidence of heart attack); improved memory, sleep, and sex; and lower incidence of Alzheimer's dementia. Estrogen can be taken daily as a pill by mouth or by way of a skin patch applied weekly.

One of the risks to women taking estrogen is increased incidence of cancer of the uterus. This risk can be reduced by taking another hormone, progestogen, either intermittently or as a small dose every day. (There are now several different effective regimens.) Every woman on estrogen replacement therapy who still has her uterus should take some form of progestogen.

Some studies have shown an increased incidence of breast cancer in women on hormone replacement therapy (HRT), but other studies fail to confirm this finding, so the question is still open. A history of clotting disorders is a contraindication to HRT. In general, though, I believe that the benefits of HRT far outweigh the risks for healthy postmenopausal women.

SAFE SEX

Safe sex makes sense at any age. All sexually transmitted diseases (STDs), including AIDS, are found in older age groups. Individuals at high risk for AIDS should be tested for HIV. High-risk groups include:

- Those who have had an STD
- Sexually active homosexual or bisexual men
- Users of intravenous drugs and their sexual partners
- Those who have had multiple sexual partners
- Those whose partner has had multiple sexual partners
- Those who had a blood transfusion between 1978 and 1985 and their sexual partners

STAYING INVOLVED

Advise elderly persons to:

- Value family, friends, and social and religious groups; avoid isolation, and associate with all age groups.
- Be uplifted by the enthusiasm of the young, listen to them, be a resource for them, and comfort them as needed.

VALUE ROOTS

Elders should be encouraged to explore their background and heritage and write it down—this stimulates the memory. Each human being is as unique as his or her memories.

ADVANCE DIRECTIVES

Well-considered advance directives about health care decisions can avert futile treatments and unnecessary prolongation of life in the event of severe, irreversible illness or coma: Should resuscitation be attempted in the event of death? Should feeding tubes be placed? Should intravenous fluids or antibiotics be given? Should the person be transferred to the hospital or treated in another setting? Clear instructions confer peace of mind on the caregivers and reassure them that they are following their loved one's wishes. (See Chap. 23 for more details.)

IMMUNIZATIONS

Elders should have a tetanus-diphtheria booster every 10 years or a single booster at age 65. Although tetanus is an uncommon disease, more than 60% of total cases occur in persons 60 and older.

Elderly people should have an influenza vaccination annually before the flu season starts. Those who look after seniors should also have an annual flu vaccination, for their charges' health and their own protection.

Immunocompetent elderly individuals should receive a pneumococcal vaccine once in a lifetime. Current vaccines are probably effective for up to 9 years. A second vaccination has been given to some immunocompromised patients, but because its effectiveness is not proven and it provokes more local reactions, a second vaccination should be given as indicated and not routinely.

High-risk groups should be immunized against hepatitis B. Among those at high risk are hemodialysis patients, those exposed to blood products, and those who have contact (including sexual) with carriers.

Purified protein derivative (PPD) screening for tuberculosis (TB) should be administered to those at high risk. The elderly, particularly nursing home residents, are especially vulnerable, as are the urban poor, minority populations, immigrants from countries where TB is endemic, immunocompromised persons, HIV-positive persons, and health workers exposed to any of these groups.

3
CHAPTER

Health Appraisal
for the
Robust Elder

Youth is immortal;
'Tis the elderly only grow old!
Herman Melville, *"The Wise Virgins to Madam Mirror"*

How can we help healthy elders stay healthy? One way is to do a health appraisal, which, unlike the current standard history and physical, is not solely disease-oriented. A comprehensive health appraisal addresses much more—it measures baseline daily function; advises about prevention of disease and about self health care, nutrition, and exercise; reviews in detail the use of medication and other substances; and evaluates mental and emotional health, social circumstances, and financial status. In other words, it assesses the whole person and offers customized guidelines to optimize the individual's health and function and to reduce lifestyle risks.

The initial comprehensive health appraisal can be carried out any time after the 50th birthday. (It could be carried out at age 65, when the person becomes eligible for Medicare). Thereafter, a review can be carried out when suggested by a change in the individual's status. The senior who has been through such an evaluation has probably learned the differences between normal aging changes and signs of disease, understands his or her medication regimen, and will be more confident about seeking help as soon as it is needed.

The health appraisal can begin with a self-administered questionnaire filled in at home or in the medical office (see Table 3–1 for contents of a typical questionnaire). Completion of the questionnaire is followed by a comprehensive, function-oriented physical examination (Table 3–2), which can be carried out by a nurse practitioner or physician's assistant. Baseline laboratory tests are listed in Table 3–3. The whole evaluation can then be reviewed with a geriatrician and a profile

Table 3–1. TOPICS OF SELF-ADMINISTERED QUESTIONNAIRE

The questionnaire should address the following health, functional, and social issues:

Demographics of the participant
Medical history (family and personal)
Current immunization status
Participant's evaluation of own health
Disease symptoms and signs, including falls and injury in the past 3 months
Vision assessment questions
Medications (prescription and non-prescription; allergies)
Lifestyle habits and attitudes: self health care, nutrition, social interactions, dental status, safety, exercise, tobacco use, and alcohol use (see the CAGE questions in Appendix A)
Social assessment: living situation; help with personal care; transport; contacts with others, including pets and plant care; loneliness
Life changes
Financial status
Advance directives
Depression screening questions (see Geriatric Depression Scale, Appendix B)

Table 3–2. THE FUNCTION-ORIENTED PHYSICAL EXAMINATION

A function-oriented physical examination should include the following:

Review of self-administered questionnaire plus additional information about areas of concern
Katz Activities of Daily Living (ADL) Index (see Chap. 4)
Instrumental ADL (see Chap. 4)
Tinetti Gait and Balance tests
Audiometry and Hearing Handicap Inventory for the Elderly
Vision screening
Folstein Mini-Mental State Examination
Blood pressure, measured while lying, sitting, and standing
Inspection of ears, mouth, teeth, gums, feet, skin, and mucosal surfaces
Examination of heart, lungs, and abdomen
In men, rectal examination with prostate check, if not done in last 6 months
In women, rectal and vaginal examination with Pap smear, if not done in last 6 months
Discussion of preventive health care

Table 3–3. BASELINE LABORATORY TESTS

Any or all of the following tests should be ordered if not done in the last 6 months:

Complete blood count
Random glucose
Fecal occult bloods $\times$ 3
Mammogram
Thyroid studies
Cholesterol
Urine analysis

Other tests should be ordered according to abnormal findings.

drawn up, including medical, functional, medication, and social aspects. Written recommendations can be given to the patient, with referral as desired to other health professionals and community support systems. Patients' questions are encouraged and answered throughout the process.

The goals of such an evaluation are to:

- Educate the robust senior and help him or her stay healthy.
- Screen for morbidity from physical, mental, or medication sources and treat sooner rather than later.
- Offer links with community and other support systems.

2
PART

Geriatric
Evaluation

Happiness is a by-product of function.
You are happy when you are functioning.
William Burroughs at age 78

4
CHAPTER

The Special Clinical Evaluation of the Elderly

For to live is to function. That is all there is in living.
Oliver Wendell Holmes Jr. (1841–1935), *from a radio address on his 90th birthday*

A special clinical evaluation of the sick elderly patient is *essential* because aging and disease affect not just health, but function.

PEARL: Loss of function = Loss of independence

Many factors, both singly and combined, can significantly affect the aging individual:

- Physiological changes in mind and body, especially if extreme.
- Variability between individuals and within body systems. Variability increases as the years pass and can make diagnosis and management of disease and injury more difficult.
- Decreased reserve in each body system.

25

- More fragile maintenance of homeostasis and slower return to it.
- Immune system deterioration, contributing to an altered response to disease, and slower and often incomplete recovery from illness.
- Multiple pathology, which is common in the elderly. Chronic disorders that accumulate with aging can combine to cause major problems.
- Atypical presentation of acute, subacute, or chronic disease. Such presentations are common in the elderly and failure to recognize them can delay diagnosis and treatment.
- Aging alters the sensitivity to medications in many elders.
- Multiple medications. Most elderly patients use multiple prescription, nonprescription, or alternative therapies, affecting the sensitivity to each one.

COMPREHENSIVE GERIATRIC EVALUATION

One of the most important goals of a comprehensive geriatric evaluation is to identify and treat all reversible causes of disability. Disease, which is only one of the causes, must be diagnosed and treated, but maintenance or restoration of function is paramount. **PEARL: If the treatment of disease will seriously compromise function, a detailed analysis of risk versus benefit *must* be carried out, and the effect on the elder's quality of life taken into account.**

History

The history is the same as in medical assessment at any age, with the following variations:

- The older the patient, the *less* relevant the family history is to the current situation.
- The older the patient, the *more* relevant the social history is to the current situation.
- Major life events such as bereavement and hospitalization can have a significant impact on health and function. (This is true at any age.)

- Nutritional status should be assessed because this can affect health.
- Leading questions may be needed about sensitive subjects like urinary incontinence and sexual practices.
- Ask questions about the special senses: How functional are the patient's vision and hearing? Can he or she see to dial the telephone, write a check, recognize currency? Clear sensory input is needed for daily activities and optimal brain function. Deafness has sometimes been misinterpreted as dementia.
- Ask questions about any change in memory.
- Look for signs of depression. This is a treatable cause of pseudodementia and can be difficult to diagnose. Administer the Geriatric Depression Scale in Appendix B. (See also "Masked Depression" in Chap. 12.)
- Ask the CAGE questions (see Appendix A) to address alcohol use, then ask "How much do you drink each day?"

Functional Assessment

PEARL: The patient or caregiver can be questioned about daily function, but *direct observation* by a health professional of the patient carrying out activities of daily living is better. A home visit is the best way to accurately assess function, gait, and balance.

Activities of Daily Living (ADLs)

Can the patient groom, dress, eat, toilet, and walk or transfer without help? With help? Not at all? This is a simple assessment of basic skills.

Instrumental Activities of Daily Living (IADLs)

Can the patient shop, prepare food, manage finances, do housework, use the telephone, and use his or her own or public transportation safely? Without help? With help? Not at all? This assesses the ability to live independently.

Gait and Balance

Can the patient get up easily from an armless chair and walk steadily with normal gait for age, turn around, walk back, and sit down?

The patient stands with eyes closed, hands at side. How steady is he or she after a gentle push on the sternum? (Stand close and be prepared to help your patient if needed when you do this test.)

Detailed Medications Review

Review prescription, nonprescription, and alternative therapies at each visit. Have the patient bring every pill or potion that passes his or her lips. The medications check list in Appendix C is useful here. The patient can fill it out at home or while waiting to see you, and you can check it at the visit against the medicines brought. Check the expiration date on each medication.

Physical Examination

The basic physical examination is the same for elders as for younger age groups, with the following important additions:

- Take the blood pressure with the patient sitting. Have the patient stand and check the blood pressure again. Keep the patient standing, and continue the physical examination, and then recheck the blood pressure after 5 minutes. (See "Postural Hypotension" in Chap. 6.)
- Check for tender or thickened temporal arteries.
- Test vision with and without eyeglasses.
- Test hearing with and without hearing aids. Check ears for wax. If wax is present, remove it and check hearing again.

- Inspect teeth or dentures, gums, and whole oral cavity.
- Do a rectal examination on every patient.
- Do a pelvic or genital examination on every patient.
- Do mental testing on every patient. Screening tests include three-item recall and the Mini-Mental State Examination. (In practice it makes sense to start with the three-item recall. If the patient cannot do this, there is no point in wasting time doing the whole Mini-Mental test.)
- Do incontinence studies if needed (see Chap. 8).

Laboratory Studies

Basic Studies

Complete blood cell (CBC) count
Urinalysis (dipstick)
Thyroid studies
Fecal occult blood × 3
Tests for syphilis
Blood glucose

Other Tests

Electrolytes; renal function as indicated
Mammogram: depending on risk history, every 1 to 2 years until age 75
Sigmoid/colonoscopy: relate to family history of bowel disease, age of patient, previous bowel disease in patient
Pap smear if none in past 3 years
Other blood tests and investigations as clinically indicated

EVALUATION OF THE PATIENT IN A SKILLED NURSING FACILITY (SNF)

Inhabitants of skilled nursing facilities (SNFs) are functionally frail. They have a collection of chronic disorders that contribute to their inability for self-care. As the population continues to age, there will be more frail elderly in the community and living in institutions. Permanent SNF residents currently represent approximately 5% of the elderly population. Almost 20% of those 65 and older will be a patient in an SNF at some time.

The two most common reasons for permanent SNF placement are:

- Loss of bladder and bowel control
- Mental deterioration with unmanageable behaviors

Skilled Nursing Facility Patients

SNF patients fall into one of the following groups:

1. **Those with permanent loss of function.** These make up the majority of SNF patients. They are frail elderly with conditions such as mental disease, neurologic disorders, severe arthritis, and incontinence. Multiple pathology (for example, chronic obstructive pulmonary disease [COPD] + congestive heart failure [CHF] + diabetes mellitus [DM] + anxiety-depression) is the norm. These elders will stay in the SNF for the rest of their lives.

2. **Those with temporary loss of function.** Examples include those recovering from hip fracture, mild to moderate stroke, early COPD, resolving infections, or cancers responding to treatment. The expectation here is rehabilitation, improvement, then return home.

3. **Hospice patients.** A small number of patients enter a nursing home to die. A good SNF can give satisfactory hospice care. In some cases, nurses from the hospice team can visit the SNF and work with the staff to make this final journey as easy and symptom free as possible.

4. **Severely damaged young and middle-aged patients.** Some SNFs are licensed for subacute care and intensive rehabilitation. Most of the patients who need this kind of care are under age 65. Examples include recent road accident victims or patients with incurable neurologic diseases, some of

whom are ventilator-dependent. The family, devastated by the tragic disease or injury, usually has no idea how little time in the SNF will be paid for by their health insurance. (They may not even have health insurance.) This kind of SNF care is expensive, and the patient who does not recover quickly and cannot afford to continue paying will have to go home. Permanent disability for 2 years, if the patient is under 65 years old, is a requirement before receiving benefits under Medicare, and even then the benefits given to the disabled patient are not generous.

Planning home care for a severely disabled person should start as early as possible to prepare the family for the mammoth task ahead of them. Some families respond with kindness, love, and heroic self-sacrifice and manage to give good care. However, there is an increased incidence of divorce, depression, and other morbidity among caregivers, as well as overuse of drugs and alcohol. (The impact can be similar to the effect of caring for an Alzheimer's patient. See Chap. 10.)

The SNF staff often become attached to these patients and should be given help with their own feelings about severe injury, chronic disability, and death.

The Needs of SNF Patients

Evaluation on Admission

SNF patients need a special evaluation on admission that not only screens for physical and mental disease, but also reviews function and plans how it can be improved. The better the function, the more independent the person in any setting and the better his or her quality of life is likely to be.

PEARL: Advance directives *must* be addressed as soon as reasonable with the patient, his or her family, or both.

A form that covers essential points of the evaluation of the SNF patient is in Appendix D. It should be completed by the visiting health professional at the first assessment visit, and a plan of management developed and shared with the SNF staff.

Follow-up Evaluations

At each routine visit thereafter, the visiting health professional should review:

1. Change of condition since last visit

Is the weight stable? (What is this patient's ideal body weight? Minor fluctuations of ±2 lb are probably OK.)

Is the patient eating well?

Is bowel and bladder function unchanged?

Has the patient's function changed in any way? If so why? Look for injury, disease, or medication change.

Review vital signs and any special indicators such as blood sugars in a diabetic.

Is there a change in the mental or emotional state such as confusion, anxiety, or combativeness? If so, why? Pain in the demented patient can manifest as agitation, aggressive behavior, or hitting. Even demented patients can tell or show where they are in pain. Patience and a gentle approach are essential. A full bladder or impacted bowel can be the cause of a change.

If a patient's condition changes, always suspect a medication effect.

Always talk with the nurse who knows the patient best and read the nurses' notes.

2. Medications

Do a detailed review of medications at each visit. *Can you stop or reduce any?*

On the other hand, **PEARL: If the patient is doing well, and experiencing no side effects from medications (especially while receiving antipsychotic medications), don't change anything, even if the reviewing pharmacist suggests a taper. Use your clinical judgment here.**

If there is a new symptom, review all medications carefully.

3. Existing Disease

Manage chronic disease for *comfort and function*, with nonmedication interventions whenever possible.

Acute or subacute disease superimposed on chronic physical or mental disease can pose a difficult diagnostic problem. Remember, common disorders occur commonly. The following are the big four to look for first if the patient's mental or physical condition changes in any way:

- Pneumonia
- Urinary tract infection (UTI)
- Fecal impaction (partial or to the point of obstruction)
- Medication side effects

Don't prescribe a medication for every symptom or condition; this will poison your patient.

PEARL: At every visit,
LISTEN TO YOUR PATIENT;
LOOK AT YOUR PATIENT;
TOUCH YOUR PATIENT.

Don't be one of the doctors who zips in, signs a pile of charts, and zips out again without speaking to either patients or staff.

4. Laboratory Tests

Do not order lab tests without a good reason. (See Chap. 5.)

How to Improve Care in the SNF

The media make money from bad news, so they focus on horror stories from SNFs, much to the chagrin of the many dedicated, hard-working SNF staff members. There are clean, kind, efficient nursing homes where the patients are well cared for and treated with respect and affection. The visiting health professional can elevate the care in *any* nursing home by becoming involved, being available, visiting regularly, and giving praise where it is due. (SNF staff get more criticism than praise whether merited or not.) Nurse practitioners and physician's assistants have skills that bridge medicine and nursing, and can provide excellent SNF patient care. They are also less intimidating to staff than the often uninterested MD.

PEARL: For best results, build a team with the SNF staff.

EVALUATION OF THE
HOMEBOUND PATIENT

Hospitals and nursing homes are dangerous places: resistant organisms live there. Whenever possible, there really is no place like home in sickness or in health.

The home-care nurse is the key person in this setting, with the physician as consultant and other health professionals such as medical social workers, rehabilitation team, and dietitians involved as needed.

Home Care Patients

1. **Chronically sick people of all ages with permanent loss of function.** Examples include quadriplegics, ventilator-dependent patients, and those with incurable neurologic diseases, crippling arthritis, or dementia. These patients are a heavy burden for caregivers. (See Chap. 10.) Community recognition of the burden on the family helps to counter feelings of isolation and being overwhelmed. The importance of support systems from the hospital, SNF, community, paid organizations, national organizations, volunteers, and religious groups cannot be overstated.
2. **Those with temporary loss of function.** Examples are patients with a fractured hip or a resolving stroke. For most of these patients, rehabilitation in the familiar home setting will aid recovery. The physical or occupational therapist, together with the home-care nurse, can carry out a home safety inspection (see Chap. 14) and give valuable advice about assistive devices. Community support systems also can help.
3. **Young sick people who will get better.** An example might be a child with osteomyelitis on home IVs. A nurse visits for teaching and evaluation of the home situation and safety. Then the patient can

come to an outpatient infusion center. The child is likely to do better in the familiar home setting and in many cases can even attend school.
4. **Hospice-at-home.** See Part 6, At the End of Life.

Parts of the Evaluation of the Homebound Patient

The evaluation of the homebound patient is similar to the evaluation of the SNF patient. Function is of prime importance, with disease sought and treated where appropriate. Medications can be reviewed more thoroughly in the home than anywhere else. Teaching (such as self-management of diabetes) also is most effective in this setting, and support systems and family dynamics are best seen here.

An example of an evaluation form for a homebound patient is in Appendix E.

5
CHAPTER

Laboratory Tests in the Geriatric Patient

DIAGNOSTIC TESTING

The older the patient, the more difficult it is to interpret laboratory tests. Body system variability increases with age, and variations in diet, multiple drugs, and chronic disease accumulation add to the differences. Also, the patient's sex, weight, and posture when the sample is taken; the timing of the sample; the time since the last meal; and exercise, medications, and the use of caffeine, tobacco, and alcohol can all affect test results.

In addition, not all laboratories are created equal. Flaws in collection or handling of specimens and in equipment or its use can lead to error. It is essential to obtain the range of normal values from each laboratory to which specimens are sent. There can be variation from one laboratory to another.

Because every test in existence has false positives and false negatives, every test ordered should have a clear purpose, such as:

- To confirm a diagnosis
- To rule out or confirm disease already suspected from a good history and physical examination

- To track change
- To monitor response to therapy

The clinician should be able to describe how management of the condition will be influenced by the test result. Will it help the patient in terms of function or prognosis? Will it influence treatment? The test should be done only if these criteria are met.

Both the dollar cost to the patient and the discomfort involved should be included in the risk-benefit analysis of laboratory tests and other investigations.

"ROUTINE" TESTS

Panels of tests are sometimes ordered without a diagnostic or therapeutic plan in mind—just a vague idea of picking up some disease process. This practice is costly and of no value to either doctor or patient. If the pre-test likelihood of disease is low in an asymptomatic patient, the yield from "routine" testing will be correspondingly low. No test should be ordered without a good clinical reason. Testing is no substitute for time spent with the patient. If management of the patient's condition will not be influenced in any way by a test result, why do the test? If the clinical situation demands treatment regardless of test results, order tests only to monitor response to therapy.

The likelihood that a disease is present when a *random* abnormal test value is obtained on "routine" testing depends on the test's specificity and sensitivity and how abnormal the result is. Minimally abnormal values are likely to be associated with minimal or no disease.

In a 20-test chemistry screen, *there is a 64% chance of at least one out-of-range value in a healthy patient*. In other words, two out of three *healthy* people given this panel will have at least one abnormal test result! This confirms the dictum that more tests do not necessarily produce more clarity or diagnostic certainty, nor do they necessarily help in management of the patient.

PEARL: In any setting, inpatient or outpatient, a thorough history and physical examination followed by a few carefully chosen tests will give more useful information than a cursory examination followed by an extensive, expensive battery of laboratory tests.

LABORATORY TEST VALUES THAT MAY CHANGE WITH AGING

Alkaline Phosphatase

Alkaline phosphatase levels increase with age, osteoporosis, healing bone fracture, and many medications. Subjects with blood groups O and B may have significant amounts of intestinal alkaline phosphatase in their serum, especially after a heavy meal. This test should be done in fasting state. Suspect disease only if the level is more than 20% above the normal range.

Serum Albumin

Some studies suggest a decrease with aging, possibly related to poor diet, chronic disease, or both. Others show no change in the healthy elderly.

Glucose Tolerance

Glucose tolerance decreases with age, but there is no significant change in fasting blood glucose.

Proteinuria

A trace of proteinuria is found in 30% of healthy elderly people.

Serum Creatinine

Serum creatinine values in the elderly can be misleading because diminished clearance plus declining muscle mass can give a seemingly "normal" creatinine level. Creatinine clearance is a more useful indicator of renal function. The following formula can be used to estimate creatinine clearance:

Men: Estimated creatinine clearance

$$(mL/min) = \frac{(140 - age) \times weight\ in\ kg}{72 \times serum\ creatinine}$$

Women: Do above calculation and multiply answer by 0.85

Rheumatoid Factors in Nonarthritic Patients

Of patients older than 70 years, 10% have positive tests for rheumatoid factors without significant evidence of arthritis. The presence of these autoantibodies probably reflects the presence of chronic disease rather than a change with normal aging.

3

Disease and Injury in the Elderly

Illness is the night-side of life, a more onerous citizenship. Everyone who is born holds dual citizenship, in the kingdom of the well and in the kingdom of the sick.
Susan Sontag, *Illness as Metaphor (1978)*

6

CHAPTER

Atypical Symptoms and Signs of Disease

Disease onset in the elderly is often insidious. Symptoms and signs are more subtle than the classic presentations seen in younger patients. Physical disease can present with change in mental state, failure to thrive, loss of function, or a combination of these. Mental changes can be caused not only by brain disease itself or by physical disease but also by medications. Iatrogenic disease caused by single or multiple medications is common in the elderly. And even without major illness, a considerable loss of function may result from multiple minor disorders. Prolonged immobility, harmful at any age, can be deadly in the elderly.

The rest of this chapter discusses some symptoms and signs of disease that may be different in older patients than in younger patients.

PAIN

In patients of all ages, severe pain does not necessarily mean life-threatening disease (e.g., migraine), and serious disease need not be painful. Cancer, for example, often presents as a painless mass. **PEARL: Pain is less reliable in the elderly than in younger age groups.** In the confused elder, restlessness and agitation may be the only signs of discomfort. In the elderly in general, pain may be absent or atypical even in the presence of significant disease. The following are some examples:

- **Myocardial Infarction (MI):** The typical crushing chest, neck, and left arm pain can be absent or minimal in the elderly. MI can present with dyspnea (caused by congestive heart failure [CHF], especially in older women; CHF applies more to women than to men); confusion; syncope (possibly with falling); arrhythmia; or a combination of these. Watch out for silent MI in elders with diabetes.

- **Pneumonia** can present with confusion, fall, lassitude, and minimal or no pleuritic pain. The only sign might be a slight increase in respiratory rate, with a tinge of cyanosis at the lips, in a lethargic patient.

- **Cystitis** can present with suprapubic discomfort, confusion, and restlessness, with minimal or no dysuria.

- **Fracture** can present with weakness in the affected limb, and a change in gait (limping). Usually the injured limb is painful, but distinguishing the new pain of fracture from the chronic pain of degenerative joint disease can be difficult. If a patient has pain in a limb, examine the joints proximal and distal to the site of the pain because they could be the source of the disease that is causing the pain. Although fracture should be suspected in the frail elder, there are many other reasons for pain in a limb such as degenerative joint disease, septic arthritis, flare-up of gouty arthritis, or (very important) a metastasis from a primary cancer elsewhere in the body. Thyroid, breast, colon, lung, and prostate cancers commonly spread to bone, and pain in a limb could be the first indication of any one of these. Pathologic fracture can occur at the site of a bony metastasis.

- **Acute abdomen.** The patient may have little or no pain, fever, or increase in white blood count (WBC), even in peritonitis, perforated peptic ulcer, or perforated diverticulum. Any of these can present with confusion, lethargy, and anorexia. Perforation occurs earlier in the course of the disease in the elderly and has more serious consequences.

- **Bowel obstruction** can develop slowly, with little or no abdominal pain. It may result from constipation with fecal impaction.
- In **referred** pain, a segment can be missed. Angina caused by cardiac ischemia in the elderly may manifest by pain in the jaw only, or pain in the hand while the rest of the arm is pain free. It can help you to recognize referred pain if you remember that there may be no tender spot at the site of the pain.

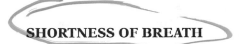

SHORTNESS OF BREATH

Shortness of breath at rest is pathologic. **PEARL: An increase in respiratory rate may be the presenting sign of significant cardiorespiratory compromise in an elderly person whose sole complaint is that he or she just does not feel well.** Look for the following causes:

Pneumonia
MI (can be silent)
CHF
Exacerbation of chronic obstructive pulmonary disease (COPD)
Pulmonary embolism
Impending septic shock
Anemia (usually produces dyspnea on exertion)

EDEMA

All the usual local and general causes can lead to edema in older people. In addition, postural edema is a common sign in the elderly and immobile. Postural edema involves swollen feet and ankles without cardiac, respiratory, or other symptoms or abnormality. It is secondary to immobility and poor circulation and is often seen in obese elders. Treatment with diuretics can be inappropriate, however, producing hypokalemia and hypotension, which can lead to falls. Caregivers and nursing home staff worry about edema, and will need reassurance if you decide that medications are not appropriate. Patients should be encouraged to lose weight (they probably won't), be more active (there are exercises that can be done in a bed or wheelchair), and elevate their feet when sitting.

BOWEL SYMPTOMS

If the usual pattern of elimination changes, with constipation, diarrhea, or alternating constipation and diarrhea, consider the following:

Cancer of the bowel
Fecal impaction with overflow incontinence
Thyroid disease
Pernicious anemia, which can present with intermittent diarrhea
Depression (often masked; see Chap. 12)
Medications (laxatives, iron, sorbitol, narcotics, antibiotics)
Dietary supplements, which can produce diarrhea
Lactose intolerance (not uncommon in the elderly)

See also Chapter 8, Constipation and Diarrhea.

DIZZINESS

Dizziness is one of the most common problems in the elderly. Ask the patient, "What do you mean by 'dizzy'?" Pause, and let the patient describe. Don't put words in his or her mouth. No matter what you suggest, he or she is likely to agree with you, and then you will never be able to get a clear picture of the symptoms.

"Dizziness" can be thought of as falling into four broad diagnostic categories:

1. **Faintness:** medication effects (hypotensives, salicylates, sedatives, antidepressants), alcohol use, cardiovascular causes, hypotension. In the elderly, watch out for:

- Postural hypotension (a drop of ≥20 mm Hg). This might only show up after 5 minutes of standing.
- Reflex hypotension with faintness and syncope, which can occur after emptying bladder or bowel.

2. **Vertigo**: usually connected in some way with the vestibular mechanism, either peripheral or central; inner ear disease; medication effects; alcohol use.
3. **Unsteadiness** without faintness or whirling: often neurological, gait disorder, peripheral neuropathy, cerebellar or other ataxia, or alcohol use. Poor balance (check for painful feet) and altered gait cause loss of confidence in movement. In some elders this leads to immobility (see Chap. 14); in others it can result in falls.
4. **"Funny feelings in the head"**: often psychological, anxiety with hyperventilation, depression-anxiety state, manipulation to gain attention and sympathy. Having the elderly patient complete the Geriatric Depression Scale (Appendix B) could help with this diagnosis. (See "Masked Depression" in Chap. 12.)

Notice that medication effects and alcohol use occur in more than one category. When they are added to other reasons for unsteadiness, falls and injury become even more likely.

PEARL: In elders who present with "dizziness," BOB! Beware Of Bleeding! Bleeding can present in this nonspecific way. The elderly do not tolerate blood loss well. You should also check for wax in the ears of every older patient with "dizziness."

TREMOR

Essential Tremor

Essential tremor is an asymmetric tremor accentuated by action. It most often affects the hands (where it may be absent at rest but present with activity), head, or voice and is common in the elderly. Its cause is unknown. There is often a positive family history, but no accompanying neurological symptoms or signs. Fatigue and emotion worsen this kind of tremor.

No treatment is needed unless the tremor interferes with function. Complete control with any therapy is unlikely. Exercise and stress reduction are worth trying. Also, alcohol temporarily suppresses the tremor, so a glass of wine before a meal can be helpful.

Beta-blockers may be used. Give up to 320 mg daily of short-acting preparation in divided doses, or long-acting preparation in a single dose given at night. Remember side effects, particularly depression.

Another possibility is primidone, given in a dosage of up to 250 mg daily, in divided doses or a single dose at night. Start with 25 mg and increase gradually. Sedation is a common side effect.

Benzodiazepines are usually not effective, and they can cause confusion and impair balance.

Carbonic anhydrase inhibitors occasionally are successful. You can try alternate-day therapy to reduce side effects.

Parkinsonian Tremor

Besides essential tremor, Parkinson's disease is the most common cause of tremor in the elderly. Unlike essential tremor, the tremor in Parkinson's is present at rest and improves with movement. It may affect limbs or the chin but not the head or voice. The tremor of the hands is described as **pill rolling**. The gait is referred to as **festinant**—shuffling with a tendency to speed up. **Cogwheel** muscular rigidity and slowness of movement (bradykinesia) are present. The patient is at high risk for falls.

The patient with Parkinson's can benefit from the services of a physical therapist or an occupational therapist, as well as from a home safety inspection (see Chap. 14) and mobility and stability aids.

Several medications are used to treat patients with Parkinson's:

- **Levodopa and carbidopa (Sinemet).** Dosage is highly variable. Use the lowest possible dose. For some patients, the regimen can be converted to a controlled-release preparation.
- **Amantadine (Symmetrel).** Give 100 mg by mouth (po) twice daily (BID) to start, increasing

slowly to up to 400 mg daily in divided doses. Side effects include postural hypotension and cognitive dysfunction.

- **Pergolide (Permax)** and **bromocriptine (Parlodel)** may help in early stages (and recent studies suggest they also may help in later stages).
- **Selegiline (Eldepryl).** This MAO (monoamine oxidase) inhibitor can be used in the early stages at a dosage of 5mg BID, the first dose in the morning and the second at lunch. Although expensive, it can delay the patient's need for levodopa-carbidopa and also minimize this drug combination's loss of efficacy.
- **Anticholinergics (Artane, Cogentin).** These drugs are less useful in the elderly than in younger patients because they have too many side effects.

Do not stop any anti-Parkinson medications abruptly. Instead, taper them slowly.

A parkinsonian tremor that compromises activities of daily living (ADLs) and does not respond to medical treatment might be helped by thalamotomy. Thalamic stimulation, similar in principle to a cardiac pacemaker, has been developed recently and is being tested in a multicenter trial. Preliminary results are favorable, with few side effects seen. However, most health insurance will not pay for experimental procedures such as this.

Cerebellar Tremor

Cerebellar tremor, also called **intention tremor,** is caused by neurological disease of the cerebellum. It is provoked by movement. No treatment is effective.

INAPPROPRIATE BODY TEMPERATURE RESPONSE

The regulation of body temperature is less efficient with aging. The fever response to even severe infection may be blunted; temperature may be increased, normal, or decreased. **PEARL: Normal temperature does**

not mean no infection. Little or no temperature response to significant infection is a bad prognostic sign.

Use a low-reading thermometer to detect hypothermia, which should suggest associated conditions such as hypothyroidism or sepsis.

Rigors (chills) are uncommon in the elderly.

INAPPROPRIATE WBC RESPONSE

The immune system becomes less efficient with aging. **PEARL: The white blood count (WBC) may increase, remain normal, or decrease in the presence of infection.** As with temperature, little or no WBC response to significant infection is a bad prognostic sign.

Elderly patients may have positive blood cultures without dramatic symptoms or signs. Keep a high index of suspicion for sepsis in any sick elder.

LOW HEMOGLOBIN

PEARL: A decrease in hemoglobin is almost the rule in advanced age and debility, but physiological aging alone does not cause it. Look for pathology. All the usual causes of low hemoglobin can affect the elderly, plus some others:

- **Bleeding.** BOB! (Beware of bleeding!) The elderly do not tolerate bleeding well and their condition can deteriorate rapidly. (See also the ABCDs of acute illness in Chap. 7.)
- **Chronic disease** (common in the elderly).
- **Chronic renal failure**.
- **Alcoholism.** Associated with alcoholism may be GI bleeding, poor nutrition, liver disease, and general neglect. Increased MCV (mean corpuscular value) can be linked with unsuspected alcohol consumption.
- **Medications**, including acetylsalicylic acid (aspirin or ASA) and nonsteroidal anti-inflammatory drugs (NSAIDs); remember nonprescription preparations.

7
CHAPTER

The Sick Elder

CHRONIC DISORDERS

Chronic disorders in the general population account for a major part of health care time and dollar expenditures. Most medical care for these disorders is given outside the hospital. An aging population means an increase in chronic morbidity, so most health providers spend a large part of their medical lives treating patients with the most common disorders, listed in Table 7–1. It is essential to know the often atypical clinical features of these disorders and how to manage them to give good care to your elderly patients.

An acute illness superimposed on a background of one or more chronic disorders is common in geriatrics, and is a diagnostic and treatment challenge. (See Table 7–2.) Multiple medications further complicate the picture. (See Chap. 6, "Masked Depression" in Chap. 12, and Chap. 18.)

ACUTE DISORDERS—THE ABCD OF ACUTE ILLNESS

Acutely ill elders differ from younger patients in several ways. Think of the **ABCD**s of acute illness:

Table 7–1. MOST COMMON CHRONIC DISORDERS IN THE ELDERLY

Arthritis
Hypertension
Cardiovascular disease
Non–insulin-dependent diabetes mellitus (NIDDM)
Orthopaedic disorders
Mental disorders
Hearing impairment
Chronic obstructive pulmonary disease (COPD)
Cataract
Other visual problems
Sinusitis

The As

Aging Itself

"Normal" aging changes, if extreme, can complicate the picture and mimic disease as well as contribute to it. (See Part 1, Normal Aging.)

Atypical Presentation of Disease

In many older people, acute illness presents in vague, nonspecific ways, with changes in mentation often the most prominent feature. (See Chaps. 6 and 9.)

Affect of Patient

Depression can present as a pseudodementia. It is said to be one of the most underdiagnosed conditions in the elderly. (See Chap. 12.)

Advance Directives

It is of great importance to know the wishes of the patient about desired intensity of treatment and resuscitation in the event of death (see Chap. 24). Families sometimes demand that "Everything must be done!"

**Table 7–2. MOST COMMON ACUTE
DISORDERS IN THE ELDERLY**

Pneumonia ± sepsis
Urinary tract infection ± sepsis
Cardiovascular disease:
   Myocardial infarction (MI)
   Congestive heart failure (CHF)
   Cerebrovascular accident (CVA)
Medication-related problems
Fractured hip, wrist, vertebrae

whether this is in the patient's best interests or not.
The caring physician will respect the patient's wishes,
if known, and help the family members to explore the
risks versus the benefits of the situation, thus avoiding
inappropriate treatment.

The Bs

Bleeding

BOB! (Beware of bleeding!) Bleeding is badly tolerated in the elderly and can lead to syncope and falls.
Rapid loss of even a small amount of blood can produce hypovolemic shock. Sclerotic blood vessels do
not retract as well as younger, elastic ones, so bleeding
can continue for longer than would be expected. Also,
tissues are more lax and significant amounts of blood
can leak into them (for example, into the thigh from a
fractured femur).

Normal aging does not cause low hemoglobin. This
condition is always pathologic. (See Chap. 6.)

Baseline

Knowledge of baseline health and function before
the incident is essential. (See Chaps. 4 and 14 for information on assessment.)

Balance

The acutely ill elder has poor balance and is at high risk for falls. Falling also can be a precursor of disease in the elderly. (See "Falls" in Chap. 8.)

Bowel and Bladder

Always check both bowel and bladder. A distended urinary bladder can overflow, giving a wrong impression of urinary incontinence. Fecal impaction can cause partial or complete bowel obstruction with liquid bowel contents leaking past, giving a wrong impression of diarrhea. Hard fecal material also can press on and occlude the urethra. (See "Constipation" in Chap. 8.)

The Cs

Change

Assess mental or physical change in the patient. If recent and sudden, it may be reversible.

Change in the environment can cause confusion in a frail elder.

Confusion

Confusion is a more common presenting feature of illness in the elderly than fever or pain. (See Chap. 9.)

Complication as Presenting Feature

A complication of underlying disease is often the presenting symptom. For example, sepsis may result from a pressure sore; breathlessness may be caused by congestive heart failure (CHF) as a result of myocardial infarction (MI); sepsis in the feet, vision-related problems, or renal failure may be caused by diabetes mellitus.

Caregivers

It can be difficult to obtain a clear history from a frail, confused, sick elderly person, so it is essential to talk with caregivers.

The Ds

Disease

Look for common disorders first, then less common. Expect multiple pathology. **PEARL: Remember the domino effect, in which many minor disorders summate to produce a sick patient. If in this situation you prescribe a medication for every disorder, you could end up poisoning your patient.** Good judgment must be used here. Treat the most significant disorders first with as simple a regimen as possible, then evaluate the risks and benefits of every other medication (e.g., side effects, impact on function) before you prescribe it.

Drugs

A detailed review of the patient's drug regimen is essential. Medication toxicity is an important cause of illness in the elderly. World studies show that 20% to 30% of acute hospital admissions in this age group are related to medication side effects. Remember, a frail elder can become toxic on "normal" medication doses.

In the elderly, expect multiple medications, both prescription and nonprescription. Also ask about alternative therapies such as herbal preparations. (See Chaps. 16 to 19.)

Dehydration

Dehydration and associated electrolyte abnormalities can be deadly. Dehydration can be a cause or an effect of illness in the elderly.

Diarrhea

Beware of spurious diarrhea in fecal impaction. Diarrhea from any cause can lead to dehydration and serious electrolyte abnormalities. (See Chap. 8.)

Discharge from Hospital

The sooner the patient is discharged from the hospital, the better! Hospitals are noisy and dangerous, and resistant organisms live there. Rehabilitation should start as soon as possible (ASAP). Function and mobility must be preserved at all costs throughout the illness. The ideal situation would be for the patient to return home ASAP with home care follow-up and as much support for the caregivers as they need. Discharge to a good nursing home is the next best situation, but resistant organisms live there too, and another move to an unfamiliar place can worsen confusion in a frail elder.

UNDERREPORTING OF ILLNESS

Illness tends to be underreported in old age as a result of several factors:

- Elders may interpret the often vague signs of disease as a result of aging, and the unaware or uninterested health care provider may reinforce this view, saying, "What do you expect at your age?"
- Elders may be suffering from depression and lack the motivation and energy to pursue other symptoms.
- Early dementia may prevent recognition of illness.
- Fear of loss of independence may suppress reporting of important but embarrassing symptoms such as urinary incontinence.

These factors, alone or combined, can delay diagnosis and treatment and further impair function. The general condition worsens and the downward spiral continues, leading to irreversible damage or even premature death.

8
CHAPTER

The Geriatric Giants: Multifactorial Clinical Syndromes

The term **Geriatric Giants** is used to describe several multifactorial disease syndromes found in the elderly:

- Failure to thrive
- Instability, gait disorders, and falls
- Pressure sores
- Urinary incontinence
- Constipation and diarrhea

Difficulty with diagnosis can arise because of the often nonspecific ways in which syndromes can appear. Regarding them as giants is well justified because of the large numbers of elderly people whom they make ill and nonfunctional.

FAILURE TO THRIVE

Lassitude with anorexia and eventual weight loss can be caused by physical or mental disease or by medication.

Gastrointestinal Tract Causes

- **Pathology in Gastrointestinal Tract (GIT).** Peptic ulcer, neoplasm.
- **Malabsorption syndrome.** Bowel symptoms may be minimal. Think of this when there is a history of gastrectomy.

General Causes

- **Any acute infection or inflammation.**
- **Chronic disease.** Usually multiple disorders; renal failure or liver dysfunction is common.
- **Medications**, single or multiple.
- **Alcohol** overuse.
- **Diabetes mellitus (DM).** In the elderly, this commonly presents with a complication—neurological, vascular, eyes, feet. (See Chap. 18.)
- **Thyroid disease.**
  - Thyrotoxicosis: weight loss may be slight; may start with signs in the cardiovascular system, confusion. "Apathetic" hyperthyroidism can mimic hypothyroidism.
  - Hypothyroidism: can start with confusion, depression, paranoia (myxedema madness).
- **Pernicious anemia.** Atrophic gastritis can produce anorexia.
- **Liver dysfunction.**
- **Electrolyte abnormalities.**
  - Hypokalemia: often medication-induced. Can occur during initial treatment of pernicious anemia.
  - Hypercalcemia: found in bronchial carcinoma; bony metastases from primary tumor in lung, breast, colon, prostate, thyroid; hyperparathyroidism.
  - Uremia.
- **Terminal disease.** It is usual for the dying patient to be anorexic and fail to thrive. These symptoms

are a prelude to death. Forced feeding can cause serious discomfort. The caregivers might need help from health care professionals to come to terms with this. (See Chaps. 20 to 24.)

- **Extreme old age.** Comments about forced feeding also apply to these patients.

Mental Causes

- **Depression**
- **Dementia**

Medications as a Cause

- Any **single medication or combination of medications**, either prescription, nonprescription, or both. (See Chaps. 16 to 19.)

INSTABILITY, GAIT DISORDERS, AND FALLS

Approximately one-third of community-dwelling elderly people fall each year, with substantial subsequent mortality and morbidity. Fractures (hip and wrist the most common) occur in 5% to 10%; 30% to 40% suffer soft-tissue injuries. Less common results include subdural hematoma (which can result from seemingly trivial injury) and hypothermia. (In all cases of hypothermia, think of associated conditions such as hypothyroidism and sepsis. See Chap. 6.) Figures for institutionalized elderly people are significantly higher; more than two-thirds of them fall each year.

Most falls have multifactorial causes. Many can be prevented. Prevention of osteoporosis is crucial because in this condition fracture can result from trivial injury or seemingly spontaneously—the bone breaks, then the person falls. A patient can fall or slide out of a wheelchair and break a bone.

Post-Fall Syndrome

Post-fall syndrome refers to a loss of confidence and anxiety about further falls, leading to immobility, which in turn can result in urinary incontinence, pressure sores, pneumonia, loss of independence, and eventually premature, dysfunctional death. (See "Avoiding Destructive Immobility" in Chap. 14.)

Causes of Abnormal Gait and Instability

Abnormal gait and instability resulting in falls can arise from one or more of the following:

- **Physiological aging changes**
  - Deterioration of mechanisms of posture, gait, and balance, with associated muscle weakness and stiffness
  - Decreased vision and hearing (Distant vision is important in balance.)

- **Pain**
  - Bunions, corns, calluses
  - Badly fitting shoes
  - Degenerative joint disease (DJD)
  - Undiagnosed fracture (Painful stress fractures without obvious trauma can occur in osteomalacia, itself a pain-free condition.)
  - Paget's disease of tibia or femur
  - Peripheral neuropathy.

- **Stiffness or spasm** in joints or muscles
  - DJD with disorganization of hips or knees; kyphosis; scoliosis
  - Cervical spondylosis
  - Contractures in Achilles tendons
  - Contractures of knee and hip flexors
  - Spastic paralysis, which results in scissors gait
  - Parkinsonism, which produces festinant gait

- **Muscle weakness**
  - Proximal muscle weakness (seen in osteomalacia) causes waddling gait.

- Distal muscle weakness (seen in peripheral neuritis) causes foot drop and high-stepping gait.

- **Incoordination and ataxia**
  - Vestibular disease
  - Cerebellar ataxia in multiple sclerosis.
  - Peripheral neuritis from any cause
  - Subacute combined degeneration in pernicious anemia
  - Tabes dorsalis in late stages of syphilis
  - Diffuse cerebral damage in demented patients

Other Reasons for Falling

- **Unsafe environment, poor vision.** Dim lights, loose rugs, slippery floors, and cracks in sidewalks are major causes of accidents. (See "Home Safety" in Chap. 14.) Poor vision compounds the danger. The recent institution of bifocal or trifocal eyeglasses may increase chance of falls.

- **Disease precursor.**
  - Infection (pneumonia; urinary tract infection)
  - Congestive heart failure (CHF)
  - Transient ischemic attacks (TIAs), pre-stroke
  - Peripheral neuritis
  - Parkinsonism
  - Electrolyte disturbance
  - Acute confusional states
  - Chronic confusional states

- **Dizziness and vertigo.** Can lead to falls regardless of cause (see Chap. 6).

- **Medications.**
  - Sedatives
  - Tranquilizers
  - Antiseizure medications
  - Hypotensives
  - Diuretics
  - Antidepressants

- **Alcohol**

Which Elderly Are Most at Risk for Falls?

Those with:

- Decreased mobility
- Poor balance
- Impaired function (impaired ability to perform activities of daily living [ADLs] and instrumental activities of daily living [IADLs])
- Decrease in distant vision
- Hearing decrease
- Decreased back and neck flexibility
- Hip weakness; knee weakness
- Postural blood pressure change
- Low mental status score
- Low morale or depression score
- Three or more falls in the past 12 months
- Multiple medications

Management and Prevention

Medical

- Do geriatric evaluation (see Chaps. 4 and 5) with detailed description of when and where fall occurred and any associated symptoms or signs.
- Diagnose and manage existing diseases, but avoid polypharmacy.
- Provide pain relief.
- Review medications. Do a risk-versus-benefit analysis on each one (nonprescription as well as prescription medications) and eliminate where possible. Educate the patient about medications and their side effects.

Surgical

- Correct painful conditions (for example, do hip joint replacement).
- Remove cataract.

Rehabilitative

- Encourage training in balance and gait.
- Encourage exercise.
- Suggest assistive devices. Easily portable devices that provide minimal assistance (such as a cane) are best. Patients who use more intrusive devices may become too dependent on them and unable to walk without them.

Environmental

- Provide self-administered safety checklist for safety at home and abroad.
- Suggest a home safety inspection. (See Chap. 14.)
- Suggest that the patient wear an alarm device to call for help if needed.
- Be aware that a conflict might arise between safety and independence. The cooperation of patient and family is essential in attempts at fall prevention.
- If the elder is of sound mind and knows the risks but decides to stay in an unsafe environment, you must accept that decision but can encourage him or her to make it safer.

PRESSURE SORES

Pressure sores result from compression of the tissues and reduction in blood supply. This produces skin breakdown and necrosis, with destruction of the underlying supporting tissue. They occur most often over bony points in debilitated patients, usually below the waist, but can be found anywhere on the body where pressure has been applied and skin nutrition is poor.

Risk Factors

Hospital Admission

60% of pressure sores develop first in the acute-care setting.

D I P S

D Debilitation
  Disease (arteriosclerotic cardiovascular disease [ASCVD]; DM; hypotension; CHF; anemia)
  Dementia
  Drugs (particularly sedatives)
I Immobility
  Infection, systemic and localized
  Irritation of skin, friction
  Incontinence of bladder and bowel
  Inadequate nourishment (Remember, obese people can be malnourished.)
P Pressure on skin, especially over bony points
  Poor circulation
  Paralysis
S Skin aging, making it thin, inelastic, dry ("Time wounds all heels!")
  Skin nutrition and circulation decreased

Stages

I   Skin warm and red, unbroken
II Superficial, involving epidermis, dermis, or both
III Extends down to or close to underlying fascia
IV Extends down to bone, muscle, joint, tendon

Principles of Management

The existence of many remedies confirms that no single one is consistently superior. The older, frailer, and sicker the patient is, the more slowly any sore or wound will heal. In terminally ill patients, pressure sores do not heal. Keep these patients comfortable and pain free.

General

- Improve activity, mobility, general nutrition.
- Treat general disease.

- Improve urinary incontinence if possible (discussed later in this chapter). A temporary or permanent Foley catheter to keep the skin dry may be the lesser evil.
- Fecal incontinence, with soiling of the sore, must not be allowed. Good nursing is essential. For the severely debilitated, enemas for bowel emptying (either as needed or on a regular basis) might be necessary.

Local

- Relieve pressure on affected area:
  - Turn frequently (every 2 hours).
  - Use special mattresses or beds.
  - Get the patient out of bed if possible.
  - Avoid friction. Beware! Massage, if badly done, can damage deep tissues.

- Remove necrotic tissue.

- Treat infection:
  - Treat local infection locally with **antiseptic preparations**. Topical antibiotics cause allergic reactions and favor the growth of resistant bacteria.
  - **Superficial culture is worthless**. Culture from deep in the ulcer can be helpful if cellulitis subsequently develops and a systemic antibiotic is indicated.
  - Treat cellulitis or sepsis systemically.

- If the skin is broken, keep it clean and moist.
  - Apply a sterile, normal-saline wet dressing to the pressure sore every shift while the patient is awake. A normal-saline gel preparation is available and is proving useful in some cases. Because it stays moist, it needs to be applied only once daily. I do not use it if I am concerned about rapid deterioration in the pressure sore. In this case I prefer to have the nurses check it every shift.

- A water pick is useful for irrigating wounds and sores.

- In some cases, occlusive dressings can be useful. Do not use them if pus is present. They can encourage the growth of anaerobic organisms.

- Consider "old" remedies:
  - A solution of sodium bicarbonate (baking soda, 1–2 teaspoons in a cup of warm water) used as an irrigation cleanses and reduces odor.
  - One-fourth strength hydrogen peroxide is useful for cleansing when pus, serosanguineous exudate, or blood is present.

URINARY INCONTINENCE

More than 10 million Americans suffer from some form of urinary incontinence, at an annual cost to the nation of more than $19 billion. The average cost for laundry and supplies for the incontinence sufferer living in the community is over $1000 per year.

Urinary incontinence is one of the major presenting symptoms of illness in the elderly, but one of the most neglected and inadequately evaluated. Ashamed and embarrassed, many of the victims don't seek medical advice and isolate themselves from human contact. Those who do seek help from their physician often find unawareness of the disorder or indifference to it and to the major impact it has on every aspect of life. It is one of the main reasons for nursing home admission and permanent loss of independence. Pressure sores are the most common complication of urinary incontinence.

Some kinds of incontinence develop gradually, but it can occur suddenly with acute illness and resolve when the illness is treated. With a clear plan of evaluation and management, *every variety of incontinence can be either cured or improved.*

PEARL: Urinary incontinence is a symptom of underlying disease, not a disease. It is not caused by physiological aging.

Fig. 8–1 is a simplified diagram of the physiology of micturition.

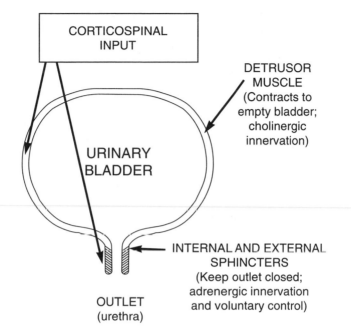

Figure 8–1. Physiology of micturition (simplified).

Causes

Transient Incontinence: **D R I P**

Incontinence of recent onset may be associated with acute disease or medications. It is often reversible if the underlying cause is found and treated (Fig. 8–1). The mnemonic DRIP can help you remember possible causes:

D   Delirium (can occur in any acute illness)
Drugs: anticholinergics, psychotropics, diuretics, alcohol, narcotics, sedatives, antihypertensive agents

R   Restricted mobility such as from degenerative joint disease, postural hypotension, gait disorders, restraints
Retention of urine with overflow, caused by drugs or prostatic hypertrophy

I Infection, inflammation, in genitourinary (GU) tract, or systemic
  Illness (any acute disorder)
  Impaction, fecal (fecal material presses on the urethra and obstructs it)
  Injury to brain (e.g., stroke)
P Polyuria, such as from DM or CHF

Asymptomatic bacteriuria, which is common in the elderly, does not usually cause incontinence.

Established Incontinence

When urinary incontinence has a longer history, it is often associated with chronic, rather than acute, disease.

Local Causes

- Weak pelvic floor muscles after childbirth or menopause
- Bladder tumor, calculus
- Outlet obstruction (prostatic hypertrophy in men, cystourethrocele in women)
- Prostatic surgery or irradiation.
- Hypermobile bladder neck (in women)
- Idiopathic detrusor underactivity (common in women)

General Causes

- Spinal cord lesion
- Autonomic neuropathy, related to DM, pernicious anemia, alcoholism
- Cerebral space-occupying lesion
- Normal-pressure hydrocephalus
- Dementia
- Depression
- Stroke
- Parkinson's disease

Classification

- **Urge.** In urge incontinence there is an inability to delay emptying the bladder after the sensation of the need to void. It is caused by detrusor instability or hyperactivity, and is the most common type of incontinence in the elderly.

- **Stress.** Stress incontinence is leakage of urine from the bladder when intra-abdominal pressure is increased, such as during laughing, coughing, or emptying the bowel. It is the most common type in women under 75 years old.
- **Overflow.** Overflow incontinence occurs when the pressure of a full bladder exceeds that of the outlet, which is partially obstructed, such as by an enlarged prostate.
- **Functional.** In this type, the urinary system is normal, but the patient either cannot reach the toilet in time because of impaired mobility, is unaware of the need to urinate (for example, in dementia), or both.

Often urinary incontinence has more than one cause. See the discussion of mixed incontinence later in this chapter.

Evaluation

PEARL: A good evaluation of incontinence takes more than one office visit.

Medical History

- **Take a complete medical history**, including obstetrical history and all previous surgeries.
- **Review all medications**, both prescription and nonprescription.
- Take a **voiding history**. The information provided helps to define the type of incontinence. This history includes questions such as the following:

  1. Do you leak urine when you cough, sneeze, or laugh?
  2. Do you wear a pad because of leaking urine?
  3. Do you ever have such a strong need to urinate that if you don't reach the toilet you will leak?
  4. How many times do you urinate during the day? (greater than 7 voids equals frequency.)

5. How many times do you urinate during the night?
6. Do you experience pain or discomfort when you urinate?
7. Do you have to strain to empty your bladder?
8. After urinating, do you feel there is still urine in your bladder?
9. How would you describe your urinary stream?

Physical Examination

- **Do a complete physical.** Focus on the abdominal, pelvic, and neurological examinations. Look for distended bladder, enlarged prostate, uterine prolapse, atrophic vaginitis, or cystocele. Test for voluntary control of the anal sphincter, perineal sensation, and fecal impaction.
- **Observe the patient voiding.** There is no substitute for this valuable observation. To overcome embarrassment, take time to explain the importance of this observation to the patient.
- Do mental testing and functional assessment.

Voiding Record

Ask the patient or caregiver to keep a voiding record for 72 hours. Information is recorded every 2 hours. (The patient does not need to void every 2 hours.) Review the record with the patient or caregiver at the next visit. This record gives supporting evidence of the type of incontinence. An example of a filled-in voiding record appears in Table 8–1. Quiz yourself—What type of incontinence does it suggest?

Investigations

- Blood urea nitrogen (BUN), creatinine, electrolytes, glucose, calcium.
- Urinalysis, with culture and sensitivity if indicated.
- Postvoid residual volume from catheterization or ultrasound (50 mL or more is significant).
- Cystometry (an easy office procedure that measures bladder function).

Table 8–1. EXAMPLE OF A
VOIDING RECORD

Time	Wet/ Dry*	Volume (mL)	Comments
8.00	W	30	On way to bathroom.
10.00	D	150	Voided before going out.
12.00	D		
14.00	W	180	Caught short, didn't reach bathroom.
16.00	D		

*Wet means incontinent.

- Cytology and cystoscopy if clinically indicated (for example, history of smoking, finding of sterile hematuria).
- Other urodynamic studies are of limited value in the elderly.

Remediable physical and mental disease should be sought and treated. Even irreversible disease, once diagnosed, can be helped.

Management

Table 8–2 summarizes the management of urinary incontinence. When giving the elderly any of the medications mentioned, either singly or in combination, start with the lowest dose, titrate up slowly, and watch for side effects.

Urge Incontinence

Urge incontinence is characterized by detrusor hyperactivity or instability. Patients have a frequent desire to void, frequent voiding, and cannot hold urine in the bladder for any length of time. The goal of treatment is to increase bladder capacity and decrease the number of voidings, both voluntary and involuntary. Try bladder training first, then medications if necessary.

Table 8–2. SUMMARY OF MANAGEMENT OF URINARY INCONTINENCE

Type	Comments	Goals	Management
Urge	Commonest type in elderly Detrusor hyperactivity/instability	Increase bladder capacity. Decrease number of voids.	Bladder training Kegel's exercises Medications: Anticholinergics, antispasmodics, oxybutynin, calcium-channel blockers, imipramine
Stress	Commonest type in women <75 years old	Increase urethral pressure. Thicken urethral mucosa. Strengthen pelvic floor muscles.	Bladder training Kegel's exercises Medications: Hormone replacement therapy (women), alpha-adrenergic agonists, imipramine Surgery Collagen injection

Overflow	Outlet obstructed	Relieve obstruction.	Surgery Dilation Medications: hormone replacement therapy (women), alpha-adrenergic blockers. Avoid anticholinergics.
	Underactive detrusor	Reduce residual volume. Prevent urosepsis. Avoid hydronephrosis.	Decompression Augmented voiding techniques Medications: Alpha-adrenergic blockers, cholinergic stimulants
Functional	Can't get to toilet in time, and/or unaware of need to urinate Immobilized by restraints Medication-related	Improve general function.	Bladder training. Move toilet/commode closer. Bedside urinal. Review general health. Review medications.

Bladder Training

Bladder training works well in motivated, nondemented patients. Even demented patients may have some degree of success. Keep a voiding record and refer to it. For example, if there is leakage at 2 hours, start by having the patient empty the bladder completely every hour, whether it feels full or not. The aim of the program is to increase the interval between bladder emptying by 30 minutes every 3 to 5 days until urine can be held for 3 to 4 hours without leakage or need to void. Combining this with Kegel's exercises gives even better results over the long term. An exercise program for total body tone-up is an ideal adjunct.

Medications

Comorbidity and other medications that the patient is taking influence the choice of drug. Monitor for side effects, urinary retention, and renal function.

- Propantheline (15–120 mg/day in 3 or 4 divided doses). This is an anticholinergic that increases bladder capacity.
- Flavoxate (Urispas) (300–500 mg/day in 3 or 4 divided doses). This is an antispasmodic, which inhibits contraction of bladder smooth muscle.
- Oxybutynin (Ditropan) (2.5–20 mg/day in divided doses, twice daily [BID] to four times daily [QID]). This has anticholinergic effects and relaxes smooth muscle.
- Calcium channel blockers (same doses as for cardiac indications)
- Imipramine (start with 10 mg three times daily [TID] and gradually increase to 25 mg TID). This has a complex action on the bladder, combining anticholinergic and alpha-adrenergic agonist effects. It can be useful alone or in low-dose combination with oxybutynin.

Stress Incontinence

The goals of treatment for stress incontinence are to increase urethral pressure, thicken urethral mucosa, and strengthen the pelvic floor muscles.

Kegel's Exercises

These work in some cases of stress incontinence, but years of weak pelvic muscles cannot be strengthened overnight. Good effects are seen after several months of practice. Bladder training as described above can be helpful.

Medications

- Hormone replacement therapy (HRT).
- Alpha-adrenergic therapy (phenylpropanolamine 50–75 mg BID, ephedrine 10–25 mg TID–QID). This increases internal sphincter tone. Avoid in uncontrolled hypertension or thyroid disease. Monitor for side effects. It can be combined with HRT.
- Imipramine helps in some cases. Watch for side effects.

Surgery

Several operations and devices can give satisfactory results in carefully selected patients. Collagen injection around the urethra yields temporary improvement in some patients. Consultation with specialists in urology and gynecology is needed.

Overflow Incontinence

Overflow Incontinence Caused by Outlet Obstruction

Outlet obstruction may be caused by cystocele, bladder neck obstruction, or prostatic disorders. Symptoms associated with outlet obstruction can be caused by hypertrophy and instability of the detrusor muscle itself in response to the obstruction. Intermittent catheterization can be used for the short term, but it is not a good long-term solution. Treat the cause if possible, generally with surgery to relieve the outlet obstruction.

In women with urethral stenosis, distal urethral stricture might respond to dilation, but be sure that the detrusor is not *under*active—if it is, dilation could make the situation worse. Hormone replacement therapy (HRT) can be tried. If these measures fail, consider surgery.

Medications

- Alpha-adrenergic blockers (terazosin [Hytrin] 1–5 mg at bedtime [HS]; prazosin [Minipress] 1–2 mg BID–QID). These agents lower bladder outlet resistance, and may be tried in the least severely obstructed patients.
- Avoid anticholinergics.

Overflow Incontinence Caused by Underactive Detrusor

An underactive detrusor can result from chronic outlet obstruction, or may be idiopathic in women. Exclude disc compression and autonomic neuropathy. Review all medications.

The goals of treatment are to reduce residual volume, prevent urosepsis, and avoid hydronephrosis. Procedures include decompression with indwelling or intermittent catheterization for several weeks. Then, when obstruction has been excluded, voiding trials can be performed.

Patients can also be taught augmented voiding techniques (double voiding, suprapubic pressure, Valsalva maneuver). An indwelling urinary catheter is a last resort with an irreversibly underactive detrusor that has not responded to any of these measures or medications.

Medications

- An alpha blocker such as terazosin or prazosin might help by reducing outlet resistance.
- Cholinergic stimulants (bethanechol [Urecholine] 30–200 mg/day in divided doses). These stimulate bladder contraction and are contraindicated in outlet obstruction. In practice, they are rarely useful. Monitor the residual volume to assess effect. Watch for side effects. Do not give to any patient with peptic ulcer, thyrotoxicosis, cardiac decompensation, myocardial infarction, or bronchial asthma.

Functional Incontinence

Functional incontinence is managed by improving the patient's general function and improving access to the toilet. Review the patient's general health, treat disease, and review all medications. Help the patient to be as mobile as possible with rehabilitation, exercise, and assistive devices such as a cane. Avoid the use of restraints, both physical and chemical. Bladder training can be successful in some of these patients.

Make the toilet obvious, safe, and easily accessible. If necessary, provide a bedside commode or urinal.

Mixed Incontinence

A substantial amount of urinary incontinence is mixed. Women can have both detrusor instability and sphincter weakness, for example. Men can have detrusor instability and obstruction. Some patients have a combination of detrusor instability and impaired contractility.

The treatment of these complex disorders is surgery where indicated, and small-dose combination therapy with anticholinergics, bladder relaxants, and alpha-agonists. Imipramine, with its combined anticholinergic and alpha-adrenergic effects, can be helpful in this situation. In women, HRT of at least 0.625 mg estrogen by mouth (or the equivalent transdermally) is worth trying. HRT can be used in addition to the other medications.

Always keep in mind the risk of urinary retention when bladder relaxants are used.

Other General Measures

Certain measures apply to patients with all types of urinary incontinence:

- **Adult diapers and protective undergarments.** If all else fails, these can be useful, especially the ones that stay dry next to the skin, but they are expensive.
- Use of a **Foley catheter** to keep the patient dry (for example, to heal a pressure sore in a bedridden, incontinent SNF patient). This can be the least of evils.
- Many **support groups** are available and offer detailed descriptions of some of the methods of treatment mentioned here. These groups are helpful for both patients and caregivers.

Ideas to Remember

You should remember several important points about urinary incontinence:

- It is not part of normal aging.
- It is a symptom, not a disease.
- All kinds can be helped, and some can be cured.
- A good evaluation cannot be done in one visit.
- The family doctor can manage two-thirds of these patients successfully.

CONSTIPATION AND DIARRHEA

Constipation

Constipation is common in elderly people. ("Not so much a symptom, more a way of life!") Many seniors are obsessed with having a daily bowel movement (fears of auto-toxicity), but the range of normal at any age is from 3 times per day to 3 times per week. Chronic laxative abuse is common.

Causes

- Altered bowel motility with aging, with or without weak abdominal muscles
- Bowel disease such as diverticulitis or neoplasm, or painful conditions of the anus or rectum (such as anal fissure or hemorrhoids), which inhibit defecation
- Immobility and inactivity; bed rest
- Diet low in fiber and fluids
- Dehydration (look for the cause; it could be medication related)
- Anorexia (look for the cause)
- Systemic disease (e.g., hypothyroidism, uremia, diabetes, hypercalcemia)
- Mental disorder (e.g., dementia, depression)
- Medications (any with anticholinergic effects, codeine and other narcotics, aluminum hydroxide, iron, antidepressants)

History and Examination

Perform a thorough history and physical examination. Ask about a family history of bowel cancer. **PEARL: Always do a rectal examination in a patient with constipation.**

Any persistent change in bowel function in an otherwise healthy person at any age must be thoroughly investigated. Similarly, bleeding from the bowel must be thoroughly investigated. Don't accept hemorrhoids as the sole source of bleeding. Rule out pathology higher up in the bowel. Have a high index of suspicion for bowel cancer. Most cancers of the bowel grow slowly and spread late, so there is a window of opportunity when cure is possible.

Management

If mental or physical disease has been excluded, all medications have been reviewed, and the sluggish bowel function is found to be caused by bad habits, the following steps should be implemented:

- Increase daily fluid intake, especially in hot weather. One glass of water with each meal and one between meals can be managed by most robust elderly people and is easy to remember.
- Increase daily fiber intake. Use bran (2 tablespoons daily), or Metamucil (the patient must be able to drink plenty of fluid because Metamucil can set into a solid mass without it), or "Power Pudding" (Table 8–3).
- Establish a regular time for emptying the bowel. After breakfast is best, to take advantage of the physiological gastrocolic reflex.
- Increase mobility as much as possible. Encourage a daily walk, swimming, gardening, or daily exercises for patients who are in a wheelchair or bedridden.
- Use a daily stool softener if indicated.
- Use a laxative at bedtime and a daily suppository to establish a routine, then reduce both to the lowest possible usage. See the "3-Day Cleanout" in Table 8–4.

Table 8–3. "POWER PUDDING"

Mix the following ingredients and take 2 to 3 tablespoons
twice daily.
   2 cups miller's bran
   2 cups applesauce
   1 cup unsweetened prune juice
Store it in the refrigerator. Power Pudding is a good source
of fiber as well as a colonic stimulant. It is easy to
prepare, reasonably palatable, and inexpensive.

- Use Fleet's enema or a soap-and-water enema as needed to clean out the bowel, then use as infrequently as possible. Phosphate enemas must be used with great care—they are hypertonic. Oil enemas can be used to soften hard, impacted stool.
- Manual removal of hard fecal material is sometimes necessary.

Fecal Impaction

Fecal impaction is usually seen only in frail, immobile patients, regardless of age. It seldom happens when nursing care is vigilant. It can cause partial or total bowel obstruction. Presenting symptoms in the elderly can be anorexia, vomiting, confusion, and fecal incontinence as a result of soft stool leaking past the hard mass and giving the impression of diarrhea. **PEARL: If an anti-diarrheal is given to a patient with fecal impaction, the results can be deadly.**

Table 8–4. THREE-DAY CLEANOUT*

Day 1—Dulcolax tablet orally at bedtime (HS)
Day 2—Dulcolax suppository in the morning
Day 3—Fleet's enema in the morning

*Can be repeated twice more if needed.

Always do a rectal examination. Hard fecal material needs careful manual removal after softening with an oil enema, then establishment of a routine as already described. Even soft fecal material can cause impaction in the frail elder who has difficulty evacuating the bowel.

Diarrhea

Diarrhea can give rise to serious dehydration, electrolyte imbalance, and debility, especially in the frail elderly. All the usual causes of diarrhea can affect elderly people. Most cases are linked to diet and are self-limiting.

Think of the following in older patients:

- Diarrhea alternating with constipation can be a sign of bowel cancer.
- Intermittent diarrhea can occur in pernicious anemia.
- Fecal impaction with leakage of bowel contents past it must be ruled out.
- Medications should be reviewed. Is the diarrhea related to antibiotics? Iron? Laxative abuse?
- Diarrhea can be caused by magnesium trisilicate in antacids and sorbitol sweetener in numerous other preparations.
- Malabsorption syndrome can develop for the first time in this age group and appear with episodes of diarrhea.

9

CHAPTER

Confusion Syndromes

Confusion syndromes take three major clinical forms:

- Acute confusion, or delirium (potentially reversible).
- Chronic confusion, found in the dementias (most often irreversible).
- Delirium superimposed on an already existing dementia. The patient's condition can be improved by quickly making the diagnosis and treating the delirium.

ACUTE CONFUSION: DELIRIUM

Delirium, or acute confusion, is a more common presenting feature of illness in the elderly than either fever or pain. Like a seizure in an infant, it can be the result of disease in the brain itself or elsewhere in the body. Delirium can be reversed if the underlying cause is found and treated in time, but mortality rates for hospitalized, delirious elders can be as high as 30%, even when a diagnosis is made and treatment started. Although delirium can occur in previously healthy elders, pre-existing organic brain disease favors its development, and many of the patients who have delirium subsequently develop dementia—some soon after, others months or years later.

The onset of delirium is acute and the patient looks sick. **PEARL: Delirium is a medical emergency and should be treated as such.**

It is easy to identify delirium in a previously normal elder, but more difficult when it is superimposed on an existing dementia. **PEARL: One of the most valuable clinical signs in this situation is that the demented patient who previously paid attention to questions but gave inappropriate answers *now does not pay attention.*** (See Table 9–1).

Causes of Delirium

Causes of delirium can be physical, mental, metabolic, medication-related, or a combination of these. **PEARL: Delirium is often multifactorial, and in the frail elder several seemingly minor disorders can combine to produce a sick patient.** The mnemonic ICM (I See 'Em!) can help you remember the most common causes.

I Infection (pneumonia, urinary tract, sepsis)
    Injury (remember subdural hemorrhage)
    Intoxication (alcohol)
C Cerebrovascular accident
    Congestive heart failure (CHF)
    Cerebral anoxia
M Medications (individual or multiple, prescription or nonprescription)
    Metabolic (dehydration, electrolyte imbalance, hypoglycemia)
    Myocardial infarction (MI)

Evaluation of the Patient with Delirium

If there are caregivers, ask them for a detailed description of the onset, nature, and duration of the illness and previous health and function. The patient is unlikely to be able to give you this information, but many delirious or demented patients can indicate the site of discomfort if you take time and listen. A detailed review of medications is next, followed by a

Table 9–1. DIFFERENCES BETWEEN DELIRIUM AND DEMENTIA

Factor	Delirium	Dementia
Onset	Sudden	Gradual
Duration	Brief (hours to days)	Long (months to years)
Level of consciousness	Fluctuates throughout day, lethargic, somnolent during day	Unaffected
Motor signs	Tremor, myoclonus, ataxia, hyperactivity	None until late
Speech	Incoherent	Normal
Language	Vocabulary usual for patient, but frequent use of wrong words	Impoverished, and worsens as disorder progresses
Memory	Impaired	Impaired
Attention	Impaired, fluctuates	Normal
Perception	Hallucinations common	Hallucinations uncommon
Mood	Fearful, suspicious, irritable	Fearful, suspicious, irritable, normal affect; depressed early in disorder
Sleep	Disturbances common	Disturbances common
General condition	Patient looks sick	Patient looks healthy
Clinical course	Fluctuates over short term	Stable over short term

thorough physical examination, with laboratory tests ordered based on the clinical findings. (But remember, an elderly patient can be seriously ill but have normal or minimally abnormal lab values, so for sick elders you must put more weight on the clinical condition of the patient than on lab tests.) These steps should show the underlying cause and allow treatment to start promptly.

CHRONIC CONFUSION: THE DEMENTIAS

The term **dementia** refers to an acquired, progressive impairment of intellectual abilities characterized by multiple cognitive deficits. Memory, language, visual-spatial function, calculation, and abstract reasoning are all adversely affected, and social and occupational function deteriorates as the disorder progresses. (See also the beginning of Chap. 10.)

Although the most common cause of chronic confusion in the elderly is Alzheimer's dementia, potentially treatable pseudodementias account for 15% to 35% of cases. An underlying cause should be sought in every confused patient because, whether the confusion is reversible or not, prompt, accurate diagnosis allows the patient and caregivers to plan for the impact of the disease on their lives. Also, early diagnosis of even irreversible dementias allows various therapies and behavior modifications to be tried, some of which might improve the patient's general condition and even slow the deterioration.

Potentially treatable causes of confusion in elderly patients can be recalled using the mnemonic DEMENTIA:

D   Dehydration
      Depression (see Chap. 12)
E   Endocrine (thyroid disease)
      Environment:
          Change or new environment
          Cold exposure (hypothermia)
          Hot weather (hyperthermia)
      Electrolyte disturbances

M Medications
     Metabolic (diabetes mellitus, hypokalemia, dehydration, uremia)
E Eye and ear problems
N Nutritional deficiencies (e.g., deficiency of vitamin B_{12}, folic acid, or folate can damage the nervous system)
     Normal pressure hydrocephalus
     Neurosyphilis
T Tumor (primary or secondary)
     Trauma
I Infection (respiratory system, urinary tract, sepsis)
     Impaction (fecal)
     Ischemia (MI, stroke, embolism)
     Insomnia
A Anemia (deficiency of vitamin B_{12} or folate)
     Anoxia (CHF, respiratory failure)
     Alcoholism
     Anesthetic

DELIRIUM SUPERIMPOSED ON DEMENTIA

It can be difficult to diagnose delirium in a demented patient; the signs and symptoms in the patient are seldom as clear as those presented in textbooks. Table 9–1 offers clues to assist you. It helps if you know your patient so that you can detect subtle changes in condition. Observant, interested caregivers also help; listen to them if they express concern.

IRREVERSIBLE DEMENTIAS

Some types of dementia are irreversible. They are discussed more fully in Chaps. 10 and 11. They include:

- Alzheimer's dementia
- Multi-infarct dementia

- Pick's dementia
- Creutzfeldt-Jakob disease
- Huntington's disease

Irreversible dementias also accompany some cases of chronic disease, usually late in the course. Diseases that may progress in this way include:

- Parkinson's disease
- Amyotrophic lateral sclerosis (ALS)
- AIDS

EVALUATION OF THE PATIENT WITH CHRONIC CONFUSION

The dementing diseases have a more gradual onset than delirium, so the patient usually comes to the doctor for the first time, or is brought by his or her family, after several weeks or even months of changes in brain function. PEARL: The first thought in every case should be whether there is an underlying, remediable cause. Next, the following points should be considered because, alone or combined, they can contribute to mental deconditioning and deterioration:

- What are the individual's expectations of changes in memory with aging? If he or she expects deterioration with age, it will probably happen. Slower retrieval of information is the most constant change with normal aging, but many elderly stay clear in their minds until death.
- Has concentration decreased? Concentration is a habit that can be lost or acquired according to circumstances and expectations. Remember the difficulty in college of getting back into the habit of studying after a long summer vacation?
- Is decreased motor function a contributing factor? The isolation it can cause can make all aspects of mental health worse.
- Is sensory input distorted or decreased? This problem makes communication more difficult and can eventually impair brain function. Some deaf patients are erroneously labeled demented.

- **Emotional and psychological factors** (stress, fatigue, anxiety, grief) can temporarily impair memory and concentration.
- **Depression** can impair memory and concentration. Masked and agitated depression can be difficult to diagnose. (See Chap. 12.)
- **Systemic illness** can impair an elderly person's cognition.
- Is the change related to **medication?** This is one of the most common reasons for an altered mental state.

It is important not only to rule out treatable disease, but also to be conversant with the patterns and progression of the various dementing disorders. It is essential to see the patient and talk with the caregivers more than once to track changes in condition.

History

Talk with the patient and caregivers; obtain a description of the mode of onset, symptoms, and the duration and progression of the disorder. Look for the pattern the disease is taking. **PEARL: Difficulty with** *familiar* **daily activities, inability to name or use** *familiar* **objects, and getting lost in** *familiar* **places are all significant features that help to distinguish early permanent brain failure from the temporary memory lapses of** *benign forgetfulness.* This condition is seen in many otherwise healthy elders who do not experience significant deterioration over time. (Temporary memory lapses—forgetting names, losing keys—may have occurred throughout the person's life.) People with benign forgetfulness can compensate for the deficiency by making lists or using mnemonics or other memory-jogging tricks so that they suffer no significant functional impairment. **PEARL: Patients with early dementia are unable to compensate for their memory loss.**

Inquire about a history of depression or attempted suicide. (See Chap. 12.)

The presence of one or more of the risk factors associated with Alzheimer's dementia would support this diagnosis. (See Chap. 10.)

Medications Review

Review all prescription medications the patient is taking, as well as nonprescription and alternative remedies. Also look for use of alcohol or illegal drugs.

Physical Examination

Look for signs of systemic disease and treat if possible. Do a detailed neurological examination; look for localizing signs. You should also do mental screening. The Folstein Mini-Mental State Examination (Appendix F) is helpful, as is the Geriatric Depression Scale (Appendix B).

Laboratory Tests

Baseline Studies

- Complete blood count (CBC), sedimentation rate, vitamin B_{12} and folate levels (Some authorities recommend testing B_{12} and folate levels only if abnormalities are found on the CBC.)
- Tests of liver function, renal function, thyroid function
- Electrolytes, calcium, blood glucose
- Test for syphilis
- Electrocardiogram (ECG), chest x-ray, urinalysis, test for HIV

Other Studies

- MRI
- Electroencephalogram (EEG)
- Lumbar puncture
- Heavy metal screen (if indicated by history and clinical findings)

If the clinical picture, laboratory tests, and observation of the patient over a month or so suggest a progressive dementing disorder, a CT scan should be done to rule out some less common but remediable conditions such as normal pressure hydrocephalus.

REFERRALS

Depending on the results of the evaluation, some patients will need to be referred to a neurologist, some to a psychiatrist, and some to an Alzheimer's diagnostic center.

For management of the patient with cognitive impairment, see Chapter 10.

10
CHAPTER

Alzheimer's Dementia

I tell you naught for your comfort,
Yea, naught for your desire,
Save that the sky grows darker yet
And the sea rises higher.
G. K. Chesterton (1874–1936), *Ballad of the White Horse*

Four million Americans suffer from Alzheimer's dementia (AD). The cost to the economy is close to $100 billion annually. As people live longer, the number affected will grow because incidence of the disease increases with age.

The average length of survival after diagnosis is 8 years, but it can be as short as 2 years or longer than 10 years. The faster the disease progresses, the shorter the life span, although it is still usually years from the time of diagnosis.

The death of brain cells produces insidious and progressive worsening of memory. As memory deteriorates, every thought, word, and daily activity is affected. Language use deteriorates, as well as the ability to plan, organize, and think abstractly. Personality can change for the worse, with unpredictable mood swings and rages. Depression is common in the early stages, but less likely in the later stages as awareness of impairment diminishes. In the terminal stages, the victim is bedridden and rigid with limbs flexed and is incapable of any self-care. The time, money, and emotional and health costs involved in the care of a patient with AD are considerable, and almost the entire burden is borne by the family.

DIAGNOSIS OF ALZHEIMER'S DEMENTIA

There is currently no specific laboratory test to confirm the diagnosis of AD. Diagnosis is made by investigating the patient for other reasons for the symptoms (see Chap. 9 for potentially treatable causes of chronic confusion), and by recognition of the distinctive pattern of the disease by a geriatrician. An experienced clinician has a better than 90% likelihood of reaching a correct conclusion—pretty good odds.

Although many research programs are currently investigating the use of noninvasive techniques such as MRI to diagnose AD, the only certain method is brain biopsy after death, and even this does not give a definitive answer in every case. (For details of how to diagnose AD clinically, see Evaluation of the Patient with Chronic Confusion in Chap. 9.)

FACTORS ASSOCIATED WITH ALZHEIMER'S DEMENTIA

The cause of AD is as yet unknown and is likely to be multifactorial. Studies have focused on many factors that have been statistically linked with AD.

Factors Associated with an Increased Incidence of Alzheimer's Dementia

Aging

The risk of AD increases progressively with age:
Less than 60 years: 1% risk

60 to 65 years: 3% risk
65 to 70 years: 6% risk
70 to 75 years: 12% risk
75 to 80 years: 24% risk
Over 80 years: 1 in 5 has AD (but 4 in 5 do not)

Some studies suggest that after age 85, among those who have remained free of the disorder, the chances of developing AD may *decrease*.

Genetic Influences

Approximately half of AD cases are genetic and half are sporadic. There is mounting evidence to support the genetic component of AD. A gene has been identified that is associated with the onset of AD after age 65. AD in younger age groups is known to be genetically determined, linked with chromosome 21. Of individuals with Down syndrome, virtually all who survive past age 40 develop AD.

The apolipoprotein E (Apo E) gene exists in E2, E3, and E4 forms. If E4 is inherited from both parents, the offspring are most susceptible to AD and most likely to show symptoms by age 70. (But not all with E4/E4 get AD.) Those with E3/E4 inheritance have increased risk of AD, with an average age of onset of 77 years. Those inheriting E3/E3 are less likely to develop AD, with average age of onset at 85 years. (E3/E3 is the most common form of the gene). Those inheriting the E2 form are least likely to develop AD, and if they do, the onset will be after 90 years of age.

Family History

Epidemiologic studies suggest that those who have a first-degree blood relative with AD have 3 to 4 times the average lifetime risk of developing the disease at any given age.

Head Injury with Unconsciousness

Some studies suggest that incurring a head injury with unconsciousness triples the lifetime risk.

Female Sex

Because in most industrialized countries more women than men survive after 65, there are more women with AD. The significance of sex is not yet clear.

Factors Associated with a Decreased Incidence of Alzheimer's Dementia

Hormonal Effects

AD occurs less often in postmenopausal women who are receiving hormone replacement therapy.

Education

AD occurs less often in the highly educated, but they are not immune from it.

Recent studies suggest a lower incidence of AD in those whose use of their own language is particularly rich and varied (implying a large vocabulary).

Anti-inflammatory Medications

At least nine published studies have shown a low incidence of AD in patients taking long-term anti-inflammatory drugs such as indomethacin (Indocin), compared with age-matched controls. One study was of 50 elderly twin pairs, where one in each pair had AD. The only significant differentiating factor was the taking of anti-inflammatory drugs by the spared twin. The suggested reason for these findings is that the brain, in a disordered immune response, destroys its own cells and anti-inflammatory drugs dampen this response. Unfortunately, nonsteroidal anti-inflammatory drugs (NSAIDs) have significant adverse side effects in the elderly.

Factors That Might Contribute to the Development of Alzheimer's Dementia

Lipofuscin Accumulation in the Brain

The significance of this accumulation is not yet clear.

Beta Amyloid Accumulation in the Brain

The body produces different varieties of beta amyloid, with differing plaque-forming potential. Amyloid plaques are found around blood vessels in normal aging brains as well as in the brain of the patient with AD. One area of research suggests an interaction between amyloid metabolism and cholinergic function. Overproduction of a protein called transforming growth factor (TGF or beta-1), which is thought to stimulate amyloid production and deposition in the brain, is being studied in mice.

Brain Neurotransmitter Deficiencies

Deficiencies of neurotransmitters have been demonstrated in the brain of the patient with AD, but whether they are a cause or consequence of brain cell death is not yet clear. Research is being done and clinical trials are being designed involving nerve growth factor, a neurotrophin found in specific areas of the brain that is essential for the life of certain brain cells involved in memory.

Factors Probably Not Contributing to the Development of Alzheimer's Dementia

Aluminum

Currently most research does not support aluminum as a risk factor. The increased levels of aluminum in the brain of the patient with AD are thought to be a consequence of the disease rather than a cause. Aluminum is the most abundant metal in the earth's crust, so all humans are constantly exposed to it.

Slow Viruses or Prions

At one time, the "slow virus" theory was all the rage—infection, a long latent period, then destruction of brain tissue. Could this be the cause of AD? This theory was popular before "mad cow disease" and speculation about prions as the cause of Creutzfeldt-Jakob disease, which causes a much more rapidly progressive dementia. Now some theorize about prions and AD, but the connection seems unlikely.

PROBLEM BEHAVIORS THAT MAY OCCUR IN THE PATIENT WITH ALZHEIMER'S DEMENTIA

PEARL: The patient's cognition is impaired, but his or her feelings are not, and he or she is no longer capable of controlling his or her emotions. Bearing this in mind helps in understanding many of the following troublesome behaviors:

- Repetitive, purposeless activity; restlessness, pacing, and wandering.
- Repeated questioning, with the same questions asked and answered over and over.
- Shadowing of the caregiver.
- Hoarding and hiding (for example, all the towels in the house are suddenly missing).
- Suspicion and criticism of loved ones; paranoia.
- Physical aggression.
- "Sundowning" (all symptoms worsening in the evening and at night).
- Insomnia (a frequent problem).
- Sexual disorders; sexual interest can increase or decrease. Accusations of sexual infidelity against the partner are common. Inappropriate exposure of genitals can occur.
- Emptying bowel or bladder in public.
- Removing clothes or dentures in public.
- Self-neglect (common, worsening as the disease progresses).
- Delusions, illusions, and outright hallucinations (in 20% of cases).
- Mood changes; catastrophic verbal, emotional, or physical outbursts, including agitation, screaming, cursing, spitting, hostility, overt aggression, or short temper.

- Anxiety, fear, and nervousness (common).
- Depression in the early stages, decreasing as the patient becomes less self-aware.

Not all of these changes are seen in every patient with AD. Some patients remain charming throughout their increasing confusion, inspire affection in those in contact with them, and are mourned when they die.

Most patients with AD are not dangerous to themselves or others, even when they have extreme emotional outbursts. An experienced caregiver can often divert attention and change the patient's mood. It helps if a reason for problem behavior can be identified. One previously calm but grumpy skilled nursing facility (SNF) resident with AD developed sudden extreme rages, in which he hit out at anyone who approached him. An astute nurse solved this problem by observing that the outbursts occurred at mealtimes or whenever anything was near his mouth. He had developed a painful dental abscess but could not tell anyone. With sedation, a trip to an understanding dentist, and treatment under general anesthesia, he was back to his old grouchy but nonviolent self. **PEARL: If a patient with AD SUDDENLY becomes physically abusive, look for a reason.** Look for a source of pain or other discomfort, such as a full bladder or bowel, or eye or mouth problems.

MANAGEMENT OF THE PATIENT WITH ALZHEIMER'S DEMENTIA

General Management

- See the patient at regular intervals. As needed, treat intercurrent disease and talk with the caregivers.
- Educate the patient and caregivers about the disorder. Link them with support groups.
- Inform the Health Department and Department of Motor Vehicles (DMV) of the diagnosis.

Medications That Might Improve Cognition

Cholinesterase Inhibitors

- **Tacrine** (Cognex) slows but does not reverse AD. It must be given in the early stages. It has significant hepatotoxic side effects, requiring much laboratory-test monitoring, and is expensive. Other, newer cholinesterase inhibitors are preferable.
- **Donepezil** (Aricept), a newer cholinesterase inhibitor, slows the decline in early stages, and anecdotal reports suggest that it is useful in treating the agitation seen in later stages. Some workers report that it helps with sleep disturbances in AD. Its advantages include once-daily dosing, no serious side effects, a lower incidence of side effects, and a shorter time to reach a therapeutic dose than with tacrine. It is expensive, but cheaper than tacrine.
- **Metrifonate, rivastigmin (ENA-713)**, and **galantamine** are all cholinesterase inhibitors that should be available in 1999.

Other Medications

- **Vitamin E.** Some epidemiological studies suggest that high doses (800–1000 international units [IU] daily) might have a beneficial effect.
- **Selegiline** (Eldepryl). This is a monoamine oxidase inhibitor, with the usual side effects and drug interactions. Some epidemiological studies suggest a beneficial effect. (See the comments under Parkinson's Disease in Chap. 6.)
- **NSAIDs.** See the comments earlier in this chapter about anti-inflammatory drugs. Side effects can be significant in the elderly. If a trial of these medications is requested in AD, prescribe one of the less toxic drugs, such as ibuprofen or naproxen.
- **Estrogen replacement therapy.** There are many good reasons for this therapy apart from effects on AD. Feminizing side effects, however, would not be welcome in men.

• **Combination** of any of the above with each other or with cholinesterase inhibitors.

If the patient or caregivers want to try any of these more doubtful "other medications," either singly or in combination, the risks versus benefits should be discussed with them. Progression of the disease should be closely monitored in such patients; the findings could add to our knowledge of AD.

Management of Symptoms

Medications such as lorazepam (Ativan), haloperidol (Haldol), thioridazine (Mellaril), trazodone (Desyrel), buspirone (BuSpar), and risperidone (Risperdal), either alone or in combination, can be prescribed to control troublesome symptoms, but often with little success, especially in outbursts of anger or violence. **PEARL: All the drugs that alter mood can also increase mental confusion in the patient with AD and have significant extrapyramidal and anticholinergic side effects.** Beta-blockers have been used to control anxiety and agitation, but they are not very useful because of their side effects (especially depression), and minimal favorable results.

The sufferer with AD looks healthy until late in the disease, so the fact that the abnormal behavior is caused by a progressive, destructive illness is not obvious. The casual observer might not realize that the inappropriate behaviors are neither deliberate nor under the victim's control, so the patient and caregivers are denied tolerance and sympathy.

Driving

The question of whether patients with AD should drive can be a major problem in the early and intermediate stages of the disease, when the patient still feels competent to drive but the family disagrees. Disabling the patient's car so that it won't start can work if the patient is forgetful. After he or she has tried to start it a few times without success, he or she may lose interest and turn to something else. Another possibility is to replace the ignition keys with nonfunctional ones. This allows the patient to carry around a familiar bunch of keys. If strategies like these don't work, the doctor can become involved to persuade the patient of the danger to himself or herself and others. By law, the physician must notify the Department of Motor Vehicles about every case of AD diagnosed. Cancellation of the driver's license by the DMV might convince the patient of the danger in continuing to drive and divert blame from the family.

IMPACT OF ALZHEIMER'S DEMENTIA ON CAREGIVERS

Throughout America, spouses provide most care to the patient with AD. The longer the couple has been together and the more affectionate the relationship, the more tolerant the caregiver is of the problem behaviors that can develop. In recent marriages, which are usually between younger women and older men, caregivers report more distress.

Grown children in caregiver roles are more overwhelmed than spouses, and have substantial internal conflict about the role reversal. They are also caught in the center of job responsibilities, looking after their children, financial worries, and their own personal relationships.

Caregivers can experience problems in the following areas, whether the patient is at home or in a nursing home.

Conflicting Feelings

It is normal for the feelings of the caregivers to change many times throughout the course of this disease. To watch helplessly while the disease produces changes in a beloved partner is bad enough. To watch AD progress in someone for whom feelings are in conflict is worse, because guilt and resentment inevitably play a part. To be obliged to provide round-the-clock, intimate care for a previously abusive spouse or parent can destroy the physical and mental health of the caregiver.

The caregiver's feelings may not only change through the course of the disease, but also conflict within each stage, as the caregiver experiences love, anger, denial, disgust, despair, pity, guilt, frustration, embarrassment, anxiety, resentment, loneliness, isolation, and worry about finances. Caregivers may fear the familiar person who is now unfamiliar; may feel trapped, with life passing them by; and may have fears about their own illness and death, thinking, "Will this happen to me?"

Of all these emotions, anger and guilt are the most frequent. Also, it is not uncommon for family members to describe long, drawn-out grieving throughout the illness and say that after the victim's death they have no grief left, only emptiness and a feeling of relief.

Depression and Anxiety

Some studies report an incidence of depression as high as 40% to 55% in the principal caregiver. Depression is more likely if the relationship was not close, and if the caregiver refuses to view the situation realistically and acknowledge the inevitable progression of the disease. Unfavorable changes in the patient's personality hurt caregivers more than loss of memory or function.

Energy Level

The constant demands made on caregivers can make them feel exhausted, isolated, and hopeless. Help and support from others is the remedy. **PEARL: The principal caregiver of a patient with Alzheimer's dementia must have time off for rest and recovery on a regular basis.** Respite care of the patient in a nursing home should be considered for a few weeks each year if finances will permit. If this is not possible, regular visits to an Alzheimer's day care center can give the caregiver an oasis of tranquility in a busy week.

Alcohol and Drug Use

The incidence of excessive alcohol use in caregivers of chronically sick people is high, and one-third of them take other mind-altering substances such as tranquilizers. These habits increase chronic tiredness and the risk of depression and disrupt sleep. They make driving an automobile or operating machinery more hazardous.

Sleep Deprivation

Chronic fatigue increases anxiety, irritability, and frustration. Morale is lowered, overall stress increased, and loss of temper over minor events becomes more likely. The sleep-deprived are more accident prone in all settings.

Health Problems

Caregivers have an increased incidence of headache, gastrointestinal problems such as anorexia and weight loss, hypertension, and heart attacks. The immune system also functions less well, lowering resistance to infections.

Special Problems of Male Caregivers

Men are generally more reluctant than women to ask for help. They have fewer friends and support systems and are at a higher risk for alcoholism, depression, and suicide. Previous generations of men have had little or no experience in the daily intimate care of another human being. Fortunately, this situation is changing as young men find it acceptable to be more closely involved in the daily care of their children.

Family Dynamics

Family members who live far away often underestimate the day-to-day problems of caring for a patient with AD. Recent studies show that caregivers of these patients are put under more stress from siblings than from friends, and the farther away the siblings live, the more stress they put on the immediate caregivers. A family conference with the treating physician, in person or by telephone, can help; the course of the disease can be discussed and worried family members can be reassured that everything reasonable is being done for the patient.

There are many variables within every family. Is the family close or fragmented? Do they fight or cooperate? Do they communicate with each other? Is one person consistently identified as the one to blame or to carry the whole burden of responsibility in every difficult situation? How well did the patient get along with other family members in the past? Is there a history of previous psychiatric disorder in any family member? Is there a history of abuse? Has there been recent serious illness in the family? What crises have the family experienced and how did they handle them? An experienced counselor can help the family work through some of these problems.

THE ALZHEIMER'S DEMENTIA DAY CARE CENTER

AD day care centers are safe places with trained staff where patients with AD are made welcome for one or more days each week, giving the caregiver much-needed free time. A mid-morning snack and lunch are usually available. Patients with AD in the early and intermediate stages of the disease benefit from attending. In the late and terminal stages they become too disabled. The types of services offered vary, and can include medical, nutritional, nursing, rehabilitation, and social services, with emphasis on interaction with other people and behavior modification. Some centers provide transportation. Unfortunately, the costs can be high, and financial help is minimal. Some centers are supported by contributions from the community and the costs to participants are assessed on a sliding scale related to income. The nearest branch of the Alzheimer's Association can provide information.

WHEN TO PLACE THE PATIENT IN A SKILLED NURSING FACILITY

It is unwise to promise the patient with AD that he or she never will be "put away" in a skilled nursing facility (SNF). In some circumstances, doing so could be the best solution for all concerned.

There are no absolute medical or physical criteria for placement. Some of the following points might help in making this difficult decision:

- How is the behavior of the patient affecting others, including spouse, children, or grandchildren? Although patients with AD don't usually hurt other people in their angry outbursts, the outbursts can be frightening for the rest of the family, especially if the patient is physically powerful and abusive. Inappropriate sexual behavior can be troublesome, particularly around young children.
- How aware is the patient of people and surroundings? Does he or she still recognize family members? Does the patient know where he or she is?
- How safe is the situation at home? What is the risk of fire, falls, wandering out onto a busy street?
- How fit and healthy is the primary caregiver? How old is the primary caregiver?
- How much help is available from all sources, both inside and outside the family?
- What is the financial impact of paying for an SNF, perhaps for years?
- What will it cost to pay for outside help for patient care in the home? Is reliable help available?

DESIRABLE CHARACTERISTICS OF ALZHEIMER'S DEMENTIA CARE FACILITIES

When choosing an SNF or other facility to care for a patient with AD, one should look for a number of characteristics than can help with adjustment and functioning:

- Minimal noise and no murals, which can add to the patient's confusion. Gentle, soothing color used with skillful color-coding (for example, the blue strip on the wall always means the way to the bathroom).
- Toilets clearly marked and easily accessible.
- Night lights available in bedrooms.
- Railings and grab bars in hallways, bedrooms, and bathrooms to improve safety. Bed rails on high beds are bad; patients will certainly try to climb over them and be injured. Attempts to tie them down will not succeed and will add to anxiety and confusion. One solution is low beds with no bed rails, or even mattresses on the floor.
- Patients are encouraged to have familiar objects around.
- A simple, structured daily routine is planned for the patients and a variety of activities and daily exercises are available.
- The staff is specially trained in the care of patients with dementia and is updated regularly. They are friendly and willing to take time with the inhabitants. It is a good sign if a particular nurse and aide are assigned to the patient; no one person can be there all the time, but the more continuity there is, the better.
- Staff stress reduction programs and counseling are available at regular intervals and as needed.
- Staff turnover is low. A high rate is a bad sign and disruptive to the patients, who respond badly to change.

LEGAL, MEDICAL, AND FINANCIAL ISSUES

Planning in Advance

Who will make legal, financial, and medical decisions when the patient is no longer able to do this? Exploring the patient's wishes while understanding still exists can ease the burden on the caregivers later. Even when some mental deterioration has occurred, if the patient understands the consequences of his or her actions, legally effective documents can be drawn up. There are now lawyers who specialize in this area of "Elderlaw." The Alzheimer's Association or the American Association of Retired Persons can help locate one.

A legal will is an essential document that can save time, money, and family conflict later. Financial planning in advance can ensure that the surviving caregiver is not left destitute. AD is a very expensive disease, in or out of a nursing home.

Advance Directives

A Durable Power of Attorney for Health Care and a living will (see Chap. 24) make clear the person's wishes about interventions in the terminal stages of the disease, and cardiopulmonary resuscitation (CPR) in the event of death. Issues such as the use of feeding tubes, intravenous therapy (including blood transfusion), placement on a respirator, kidney dialysis, and elective surgery need to be considered. What about treatment with antibiotics, transfer to hospital, or aggressive and invasive investigations in the late stages? These are difficult decisions for the family to make if the patient's wishes are unknown. Sometimes the doctor can help families make decisions by asking them "What would your relative want? Not what do *you* want—make that decision for yourself—but try to imagine what your relative would say if he or she could tell you."

It must be made clear to the family that because there is no cure for AD, measures such as feeding tubes simply prolong the slow death of terminal patients with AD. CPR is not justified because if the patient dies and is brought back, further deterioration is certain. It often takes many discussions with health care professionals to help the family to reach this point.

TERMINAL STAGES OF DEMENTIA

In the terminal stages of dementia, mind and personality are gone. The victim is withdrawn, does not respond meaningfully to anyone, and either does not speak or mumbles incoherently. Incontinence of bowel and bladder is usual. Seizures can occur in the late and terminal stages of the disease. If they are frequent, medications are needed for control.

Home visits by the doctor and other health care professionals can comfort the family and ensure the kindest, most rational hospice-type care for the patient until the end, treating painful conditions and avoiding transfer to hospital unless there is a good reason. Feeding tubes prolong the dying process and should not be used. Small amounts of food and fluid can be offered frequently and the mouth kept clean and moist. Intravenous therapy is not justified and the patient should have a "Do Not Resuscitate" order.

Relief is the principal feeling of caregivers after the patient's death. Guilt is commonly the next emotion— could I or should I have done more? **PEARL: It is important for survivors to be able to talk about feelings of relief and guilt, so they can move on to normal grieving.** Those who were able to keep their loved one at home throughout the illness are generally left with fewer guilt feelings than those who had to place them permanently in an institution. Alzheimer support groups can help caregivers work through these issues.

A wise, dedicated practitioner can help the family throughout this sad illness, in which cure is not yet possible, but comfort always is.

11
CHAPTER

Other Irreversible Dementias

Chronic, irreversible dementia comes in many types and has a variety of causes. (See Chap. 9.) Alzheimer's dementia (AD) is the most common type, but there are several others, some fairly common and some quite rare.

VASCULAR OR MULTI-INFARCT DEMENTIA

Diagnosis

Vascular dementia is the second most common dementia after Alzheimer's. The classic case has a history of one or more of the following: hypertension, diabetes mellitus, cardiovascular disease, peripheral vascular disease, transient ischemic attacks, stroke, or hyperlipidemia. The onset is more abrupt than in AD, and localizing neurological signs, often asymmetric, are found on physical examination. There is a steplike deterioration over time, with further episodes of illness relating to the underlying disorder (for example, myocardial infarction [MI] or repeated strokes).

Many cases are not clear cut, however, and differentiation from AD can be difficult. Finding multiple lesions on a brain CT scan or MRI is suggestive of vascular dementia, but there is no certain diagnostic test. Even autopsy may not give the answer in some cases.

Management

Unhealthy lifestyle risk factors such as smoking, obesity, excessive alcohol use, lack of exercise, and a diet high in fat should be addressed first. Underlying diseases such as hypertension and diabetes should be vigorously treated.

- If parkinsonian symptoms are prominent, anti-Parkinson's medications may be needed. (See Chap. 6.)
- Rehabilitation, assistive devices, and home safety modifications can make a positive contribution in some cases. (See Chap. 14.)
- Management of problem behaviors in patients with vascular dementia is the same as for those with AD. Other issues relating to patients with AD and their caregivers also apply to this group. (See Chap. 10.)

PICK'S DISEASE

Pick's disease is an uncommon form of dementia that is easily confused clinically with AD. Although usually sporadic, up to 20% of cases are familial. Language dysfunction is often more pronounced than in AD and memory may be preserved until late in the disease.

A distinctive appearance on a brain CT scan can help to establish the diagnosis. There is no cure, and management is the same as in AD.

CREUTZFELDT-JAKOB DISEASE (CJD)

Creutzfeldt-Jakob disease is a very rare, rapidly progressive, fatal form of dementia caused by an infectious, heat-stable, protein-like particle called a prion. The average duration of the illness is less than a year.

The peak incidence is in patients between 50 and 75 years old. There is no cure for it.

Recognition is important to avoid further transmission of the disease, which can result from contact with brain tissue at biopsy or autopsy, transplantation of tissues such as corneas, or the use of growth hormone produced from cadaver pituitary glands.

HUNTINGTON'S DISEASE

The peak incidence of onset of Huntington's disease, an uncommon, autosomal dominant dementing illness, is between the ages of 30 and 50 years, but 28% of cases occur after age 50. This disease is characterized by abnormal choreiform movements and psychiatric symptoms such as depression, aggression, and even major psychoses. There is no cure. Diagnosis is important for genetic counseling.

DEMENTIA IN OTHER DISEASES

Sometimes dementia develops late in the course of other diseases. These include Parkinson's disease, amyotrophic lateral sclerosis (ALS), and AIDS. The management of AD and related issues also apply to this group. (See Chap. 10.)

12
CHAPTER

Depression in the Elderly

O the mind, mind has mountains; cliffs of fall
Frightful, sheer, no-man-fathomed. Hold them cheap
May who ne'er hung there.
Gerard Manley Hopkins, 1844–1889, *Carrion Comfort*

These powerful words were written by a brilliant, introspective English Jesuit priest who died of complications of typhoid fever before reaching the age of 50. They express with chilling intensity and brevity not only the anguish and loneliness of mental illness, but the attitudes held by those who have never experienced it and for whom it does not exist. Growing older does not *cause* mental disease, and it is possible to live to a ripe old age and then die without having experienced significant mental abnormalities of any kind. However, levels of brain neurotransmitters change as people age. These changes can favor depression, which is said to be one of the most underdiagnosed conditions in the elderly population. It can develop for the first time late in life.

Depression at any age must be taken seriously because untreated it can lead to suicide. The highest incidence of *completed* suicides in our society is among elderly white men. Because there is no marker or test for depression at any age, the diagnosis is made on clinical grounds. Diagnosis can be difficult because of the atypical presentations in this age group. (See "Masked Depression" in Chap. 12.) At least 70% of elderly suicide victims had seen a primary care provider in the last month of life, about 40% within the last week before death.

Depression impairs function in the elderly and increases the disability caused by co-existing illnesses such as heart disease or stroke. It adversely affects family life and can increase the burden on caregivers.

VARIETIES OF DEPRESSION IN THE ELDERLY

These are the classifications that work best for me in my daily clinical practice:

- Sadness, or reactive depression
- Dysthymia
- Combined depression and anxiety
- Depression in the cognitively impaired
- Major depression
- Masked depression

Sadness, or Reactive Depression

It is normal to feel sad after misfortune and to go through some or all of the stages of grieving. (See Chap. 20.) When a beloved person or pet dies, most people never completely get over it. The sense of loss stays, but return to a full and even happy life is possible as time passes. A beloved pet can be the "significant other" for some people, and its death can produce as much grief as the loss of a human partner. (The American Veterinary Medical Association publishes an excellent leaflet called "Pet Loss and Human Emotion.")

This kind of reactive depression is common in the elderly. It responds poorly to medications, and side effects, such as mental confusion, can make the patient worse. In this form of grieving it is possible to be cheered up temporarily and there is no feeling of being worthless as a person, the opposite of what happens in major depression.

Counseling, exercise, good diet, and avoidance of excess alcohol are initial remedies. Supportive family and friends play key roles in surviving sorrow, and those with religious belief can get comfort from their faith. In some cases guilt about "unfinished business" with the dead person can prolong grieving. Encouraging survivors to talk about this can lead to some degree of resolution.

However, if this grieving process continues at an intense level for too long with worsening gloom and misery, and the victim considers suicide, professional help must be sought immediately.

Dysthymia

Dysthymia is the name given to a chronic condition between sadness and major depression. It lasts longer than sadness and has many of the features of major depression, but is less severe. Treatment with or without medications can help.

Combined Depression and Anxiety

When depression is combined with anxiety, diagnosis can be difficult because the constant physical and verbal activity often seen can mimic agitation.

If the disorder is mild, a regimen of counseling and exercise can be tried first. If the disorder does not respond to this regimen or becomes more severe, carefully chosen antidepressant medications can produce satisfactory results.

Depression in the Cognitively Impaired

Depression is common in the early stages of all the dementing diseases for obvious reasons. As the disease progresses and the patient becomes less self-aware, depression is less significant. Treatment with antidepressant medications is not useful because in many cases they increase confusion and produce other side effects. (See Table 12–1.)

Major Depression

Major depression is bigger, darker, and more destructive than sadness. Even though life can seem tranquil with no obvious reason to feel down, a wave of despair and despondency can overwhelm the victim. No one wishes or chooses to be in this drab wilderness. Major depression also can develop from a reactive depression that does not resolve.

Depression produces misery, isolation, and poor physical health and can lead to suicide attempts. One-quarter of all *completed* suicides in America are in the over-65 age group, with white men far outnumbering any other group.

It is characteristic for the victims to feel worthless, in some cases as if they are losing their minds or are on the edge of a nervous breakdown. The bleak despair that rules this disorder makes it impossible for the victims to be cheered up by anyone. A paralysis of action in major depression can make the simplest task seem impossible and death seem peaceful and inviting.

Risk Factors for Major Depression

A variety of risk factors increase a person's likelihood of developing major depression. Those with any combination of the following risk factors are at high risk for major depression and suicide.

- **Family history.** Major depression in a close blood relative means higher risk. In identical twins, if one develops this disease, the other has a 40% to 70% chance of falling victim even if the twins have been raised apart. Suicide in the family has the same predictive implications.
- **Female sex.** Until the age of 12, depression is found equally in boys and girls. After the age of 12, the incidence in girls starts to rise. In adults,

twice as many women are affected as men. Some studies have shown that later in life depression is found equally again in men and women. The incidence of depression in postmenopausal women receiving hormone replacement therapy (HRT) is being studied, as is the effect of HRT on post-menopausal women with depression. The results so far indicate a positive effect of HRT on depression.

- **Major life events.** Major events such as the following can make one more prone to major depression and suicide:

  - Recent bereavement or other major loss
  - Recent serious disease
  - Chronic disease with pain or limited function
  - Previous episode of major depression
  - Previous suicide attempt

- **Isolation.** This is not the same as being alone. People living alone can still be connected with others and enjoy their solitude. The isolated are cut off from others, either by their own choice or by circumstances. In prisons, solitary confinement is an acknowledged way of breaking the human spirit.

- **Alcohol.** Alcohol is a mild depressant and not good therapy in times of sadness. Men at all ages have fewer personal support systems than women do, and the recent widower can feel particularly lonely and isolated. A drink with friends can be pleasant and relaxing, but drinking alone is dangerous. Temporary solace from a readily available, socially acceptable bottle is treacherous. In the long run this can result in more feelings of depression, can disrupt sleep, and can permanently damage health. Symptoms of depression produced by alcohol can persist in alcoholics and heavy drinkers even during periods of abstinence.

- **Violence.** At any age, the physically, mentally, or sexually abused have a higher incidence of major depression than the rest of the population. Many men who were abused as children repeat the pattern and become abusers as adults. They are at increased risk for depression and other mental illness. Women who were abused as children are more likely to stay in the victim role (the abused) and are less likely to become abusers.

- **Aging.** The balance of brain neurotransmitters alters with aging, making depression more likely. Also, aging inevitably brings some kind of loss, such as one or more of the following:

  - Loss of significant others.
  - Loss of job (particularly difficult for men driven to high achievement).
  - Change in appearance, which in today's youth-worshipping society is interpreted as a loss.
  - Loss of financial security, which brings numerous other worries.
  - Loss of control of life.
  - Loss of control of bodily functions.
  - Loss of independence.
  - Loss of respect in a materialistic society that measures worth by income alone.
  - Loss of life—the longer the life, the closer one is to death. Lack of a personal philosophy to deal with this final loss contributes to depression.

- **Medications.** Many prescription and nonprescription medications (e.g., hypotensives [particularly beta blockers], benzodiazepines, nonsteroidal anti-inflammatory drugs [NSAIDs]) can either precipitate or worsen depression.

- **Anger.** Some psychiatrists consider all depression to be a result of unexpressed chronic anger.

Masked Depression

PEARL: If an older adult makes repeated visits to a doctor with lists of vague somatic complaints *unsupported by clinical findings*, beware! This could be a masked depression. The patient does not feel right, but grew up equating psychiatry and counseling with madness and lunatic asylums, and mental disease with moral weakness. Unable to acknowledge the possibility of a mental illness, the patient translates feelings of sadness and listlessness into more acceptable physical symptoms. The elder often actually *denies* depression, sadness, apathy, and anorexia. The primary care practitioner, who might be the first and only point of contact with the medical establishment, needs to be aware of this possible scenario. While looking carefully for organic disease, obvious and occult, the practitioner should keep masked depression on the list of possibilities. The Geriatric Depression Scale (Appendix B) is a helpful screening tool.

A feature of this kind of depression can be preoccupation with past life events, especially if the patient feels guilty about them. Focus on the present can even be lost in this situation. Memory and concentration can be sufficiently impaired to make the patient seem demented rather than depressed—an example of pseudodementia. **PEARL: If there is doubt as to whether dementia or depression is present, a trial of antidepressant medications is justified.**

Common Symptoms in Masked Depression

- Anorexia, bad taste in mouth, irritable bowel, gas or bloating
- Backache, myalgias
- Fatigue, palpitations, dizziness
- Failure to thrive
- Lack of interest, self-neglect
- Poor memory, disordered thinking
- Anhedonia (*"How weary, stale, flat and unprofitable / Seem to me all the uses of this world."* [William Shakespeare, *Hamlet*])
- Flat affect
- Agitation, anxiety
- Feelings of guilt
- Preoccupation with past life events, loss of focus on the present
- Sleep disturbances (Although common in depression at all ages, these can be difficult to distinguish from usual aging changes in sleep patterns. See Chap. 1.)

Table 12–1. ANTIDEPRESSANT MEDICATIONS IN THE ELDERLY

Medication	SIDE EFFECTS				DOSAGE (mg)		
	Sedative	Anti-cholinergic	Ortho-static	Cardio-toxic	Start	Treatment Range	Daily Regimen
Tricyclics							
Amitriptyline (Elavil)	++++	++++	+++	+++	25–50	100–300	Single dose HS, or divided doses BID
Desipramine (Norpramin)	+	++	+++	++	25–50	100–300	Single dose in a.m.
Doxepin (Sinequan)	++++	++++	++	+++	25–50	100–300	Single dose HS, BID, or TID, max. single dose 150 mg
Imipramine (Tofranil)	+++	+++	+++	+++	25–50	100–300	Single dose HS, or divided doses BID
Nortriptyline (Pamelor)	++	++	+	++	10–25	50–100	BID or TID
Protriptyline (Vivactyl)	+	+++	++	++	15	15–60	TID
Trimipramine (Surmontil)	++++	++++	+++	+++	25–50	100–300	TID

Serotonin-Specific Reuptake Inhibitors (SSRIs)

Fluoxetine (Prozac)	0	0-+	+	0	10	20–80	Single dose in a.m.
Paroxetine (Paxil)	0	0-+	+	0	10	20–60	Single dose in a.m.
Sertraline (Zoloft)	0	0-+	+	0	25	50–200	Single dose in a.m.
Others							
Amoxapine (Asendin)	+++	+++	+	+++	50	50–400	Single dose HS, or divided doses BID, TID
Bupropion (Wellbutrin)	0	+	+	+	75	75–400	BID or TID, max. single dose 150 mg
Maprotiline (Ludiomil)	+++	++	+	+	25–50	25–225	TID
Nefazodone (Serzone)	++	0-+	+	0	50	50–600	BID
Trazodone (Desyrel)	++++	0-+	+	+	50	50–400	Single dose HS, or divided doses BID, TID, with food
Venlafaxine (Effexor)	+	+	+	0	25	25–375	BID, TID
Mirtazapine (Remeron)	++	0-+	+	0	15	15–45	Single dose HS

TREATMENT OF DEPRESSION IN THE ELDERLY

Counseling, Exercise, Support from Family and Friends

The patient can be referred for counseling to a psychologist, a specially trained medical social worker or nurse, or even, in some mild cases of depression, to a knowledgeable volunteer. A minister, priest, or rabbi with experience in dealing with depression can offer considerable help to religious patients.

Any form of exercise that the patient enjoys will help. It's even better if the exercise involves interaction with other people.

Concerned family and friends can make a strongly positive contribution to the patient's general sense of well-being and can enhance the often diminished sense of self-worth.

Mild cases may respond to these measures alone. Also, reassurance from the doctor can improve the mental state of the "worried well" patient. Medications can be added in persistent mild depression or if the condition worsens.

Medications

Numerous effective antidepressant medications are available (Table 12–1). Treatment results are reasonably good in the elderly, with careful monitoring for side effects. The general rule of "Start low, go slow!" applies. (See Part 5, Medications.)

Because almost all antidepressants take weeks to lift the mood, the desired results can seem slow in coming. It is important for patients to know this so they do not lose faith and stop the treatment. A short course of rapidly acting methylphenidate (Ritalin) or dextroamphetamine can be given at the same time the chosen antidepressant is commenced. These drugs can "jump start" the most depressed failure-to-thrive patient, lift mood, improve appetite, and buy time until the chosen antidepressant has time to produce an effect.

Antidepressants must be taken for a minimum of 6 months and might even need to be continued for several years.

Sometimes the more sedating antidepressants are desirable. Given as a single dose at night, they can help the patient to sleep better. If lethargy is a feature of the depression, a more energizing and less sedating medication like desipramine should be the drug of choice.

Nortriptyline works well in the agitated, depressed patient and is preferable to a benzodiazepine, which can make cognitive changes worse.

If tricyclics are not tolerated, some of the newer selective serotonin reuptake inhibitors (SSRIs) can be tried. However, this group of medications can produce anorexia and weight loss in the elderly and may become less effective over time, necessitating a "drug holiday."

Anticholinergic effects include dry mouth, blurred vision, urinary hesitancy or retention, tachycardia, precipitation of acute-angle glaucoma, and constipation. **PEARL: The medications with the lowest anticholinergic effects always should be used.** Consider the cumulative impact on the patient of anticholinergic effects from multiple medications.

Anticholinergic effects (blurred vision) plus orthostatic effects equals unsteady gait, which can lead to falls.

Electroconvulsive Therapy

Electroconvulsive therapy (ECT) can be life-saving when used for the uncommon deep and lasting depression that does not respond to any other form of therapy or medication, or as emergency treatment for suicidal or severely malnourished, depressed patients. Desperate situations can justify desperate remedies if all others have failed and the likely outcome without treatment is death. Although there can be a period of confusion immediately after the treatment, this confusion usually clears, and some patients report *improved* memory after ECT.

13
CHAPTER

Elder Abuse

Abuse can be physical, emotional, or financial and may involve violation of rights, neglect, or self-neglect. Health practitioners are required by law to report known or suspected *physical* abuse, and they may report any other kind of abuse or neglect. Known or suspected abuse occurring in a long-term care facility must be reported to the Long Term Care Ombudsperson Coordinator or the police. Abuse occurring anywhere else must be reported to Adult Protective Services or the police. (See Chap. 15.)

People aged 75 and older, the fastest growing segment of the population, have the highest frequency of abuse in the adult population. The reported figures—4% to 10%—are low; many victims either deny abuse or do not or cannot report it. Health professionals need to be aware of this problem and have a high index of suspicion. **PEARL: Prevention of abuse by risk identification and early intervention is preferable to dealing with it after it has happened.** Because the roots of elder abuse can stem from childhood, the whole issue of family violence should be addressed and the vicious cycle of intergenerational violence broken.

RISK FACTORS FOR ELDER ABUSE

In the Elder

- Advanced age
- Female sex
- Dependence on the caregiver; compliance, passivity
- Social isolation
- Difficult behavior by the elder
- Increasing physical and mental impairment, which increases risk
- Use of alcohol or illegal drugs

In the Caregiver

- Use of alcohol or illegal drugs (found in more than 35% of abusers)
- Dementia, mental illness
- Inexperience at providing care, or reluctance to provide care
- Ignorance about the aging process
- Unrealistic expectations of the elder
- Lack of control, frequent outbursts of anger
- Blaming or hypercritical personality
- Abused as a child, or a witness to abuse
- Economic stress, financial dependence on the elder
- Social isolation, lack of support systems, no involvement outside the home

In the Family

- Overcrowding
- History of violence and past intergenerational conflict
- Conflict, lack of cohesiveness and mutual support
- Economic pressures
- Past history of abuse (the greatest risk factor for future abuse in the same setting)

SOME INDICATORS THAT
ABUSE IS OCCURRING

The following list is not comprehensive, but it gives some of the more common danger signals. **PEARL: Signed and dated diagrams of injuries, photographs of the injuries, or both are useful in documentation of abuse.**

- Injuries, bruises, or welts in various stages of healing
- Any injury that is not adequately explained
- Cuts, pinch marks, scratches, lacerations, puncture marks, or burns
- Evidence suggesting that the patient has been tied up
- Patchy absence of hair or hemorrhages on the scalp (suggest hair pulling)
- Bruising, swelling, or bleeding in external genitalia or anal area
- Dehydration and weight loss without illness-related cause
- Frequent ER visits for falls, fractures, and other injuries
- Presentation of the patient for the first time in late stages of disease (suggests neglect)
- A timid patient who looks to the caregiver before daring to answer

MANAGEMENT

Management of abuse may require any or all of the following steps. Attempt to keep to the least restrictive level possible while protecting the abused elder. A medical social worker is essential to help in this mammoth task.

- Hospitalization if indicated.
- Making the patient as functional as possible with physical therapy (PT), occupational therapy (OT), assistive devices.
- Simplifying drug regimen as much as possible.
- Regular home visits by health professionals.

- Reducing caregiver stress and isolation as much as possible; link with community resources, Meals-on-Wheels, Friendly Visitor Program.
- Encouraging respite care, using senior citizen and adult day care centers.
- Involving other family members to share the burden of care.
- Counseling the caregiver.
- Addressing mental disease and substance abuse in the caregiver. The threat of legal action may be needed before treatment will be accepted.
- Nursing home or assisted living placement of the elder if the burden of care in the home is too great, or if the elder is at significant risk.
- Conservatorship of the elder and estate.

4
PART

Rehabilitation and Resources

14
CHAPTER

Rehabilitation in Geriatrics

THE REHABILITATION TEAM

A rehabilitation team consists of a physical therapist, an occupational therapist, a communications therapist (formerly known as a speech therapist), a home-care or nursing home nurse, and a physician. These team members meet at regular intervals and design a rehabilitation program that fits the needs of the individual patient.

THE GOALS OF REHABILITATION

The goal of rehabilitation for the sick or injured elderly patient is a return to as high a level of function as possible. In any setting, the more functional the patient is, the more independent he or she can be and the better the quality of life. Knowing the former level of function is important for setting goals. For example, it would be unreasonable to expect to restore full ambulation to a nursing home resident who has been wheelchair-bound for the last 5 years. However, be optimistic as well as realistic. **PEARL: The functional status of even the frail elderly can be improved and life made sweeter.**

Avoiding Destructive Immobility

Immobility at any age is debilitating. In the elderly it is devastating and can be deadly. The sooner the patient is mobilized after any illness or injury, the better the chance of recovery. Loss of mobility can cause loss of confidence and motivation, which in turn renders the patient more immobile, and so on in a downward spiral. The elderly person can become fearful and unsteady and may need help relearning how to walk. A good rehabilitation team will try to halt the downward spiral, but encouragement from an interested medical practitioner can convince the patient and caregivers to keep working at restoring function. The physician who writes an order for rehabilitation in the chart and then does nothing more to encourage progress is falling short of ideal patient care. What the physician says is long remembered, for better or for worse. This is a heavy, but wonderful, responsibility.

The Importance of Small Gains

The importance of what might seem like small gains at every level of disability must not be underestimated. For example, the ability to walk 50 yards instead of 25 could enable the patient to reach the bathroom and allow him or her to stay at home.

HOME SAFETY AND ACCESSIBILTY

A rehabilitation team member can carry out a home safety inspection and advise the patient and caregivers about the following items:

- Throughout the home:
  - Use good lighting.
  - Eliminate loose rugs or mats.
  - Tack down the edges of all carpets.
  - Eliminate loose or trailing electrical cords.
  - Clear up clutter.
  - Install smoke alarms and check them regularly.

- Make a fire escape plan.
- Have a key in or near any deadbolt lock.
- Don't smoke (major fire risk as well as risk to health).
- Keep medications in one safe place.
- Clearly label all poisonous substances and store in one safe place.

- Kitchen:
  - Store frequently used pots and dishes within easy reach.
  - Avoid high shelves above easy reach.
  - Be very careful when using a step stool or eliminate the need to use one.
  - Use safe cooking techniques, such as turning pot handles inward.
  - Keep a flashlight handy.

- Bathroom:
  - Install grab bars in the bathroom in shower, tub, and beside the toilet.
  - Have a shower chair with nonskid feet.
  - Use a nonslip bath mat.
  - Set the water heater temperature at 120°F or lower to avoid burns.

- Bedroom:
  - Have the bed at the optimal height for getting in and out easily.
  - Have a night table to store necessities.
  - Do not keep medications at bedside (danger of repeating a dose when half asleep).
  - Have a clear pathway to bathroom, or have a bedside commode.
  - Have a light within easy reach of the bed.
  - Keep a flashlight handy.

- Stairs and hallways
  - Make sure that stair treads are nonslip.
  - Mark edges of stairs.
  - Have handrails within reach and easily visible.
  - Install light switches at top and bottom of handrail.

- Outside the house
  - Keep walkways free of clutter.
  - Check paths for uneven surfaces.
  - Keep pets secure so that they are not a threat to the patient or visitors.
  - Install adequate lighting.
  - Install handrails where needed.

Most accidents occur in or close to the home, and many could be avoided with forethought and attention to details. A home that has been made safe as described above is safe for the whole family, and will be easily accessible for the temporarily or permanently disabled.

There are catalogues full of special equipment such as prosthetics, splints, walkers, canes, and many other devices that can facilitate activities of daily living (ADLs) and instrumental activities of daily living (IADLs) and help the elderly to maintain independence.

REHABILITATION IN SPECIAL SITUATIONS

Rehabilitation of the Skilled Nursing Facility (SNF) Resident

Most people hope to improve and return to independent living after an illness, but even a nursing home resident who was previously functionally impaired and has now suffered an acute illness merits review for improvement. Patients in an SNF may function at many levels. Being fully functional and ambulatory is best; walking with a cane or walker is next best; being wheelchair-bound but able to get around and participate in activities is better than being bedridden. The bedridden patient who can move and cooperate with nurses and other caregivers is easier to look after than an immobile bedridden patient. **PEARL: Helping the patient to adapt most effectively to a permanent disability is a valuable aspect of rehabilitation at any age, in any setting.** The physician can be a key figure in encouraging this adaptation and helping it to happen.

Rehabilitation after a Stroke

Start as soon as possible after the event.

Acute Phase in Hospital

The bedridden, comatose, or semicomatose patient benefits from proper positioning and passive exercises. As the patient recovers, a program should be developed to help the patient regain as much function as possible. Physical, occupational, speech, and communications therapists should work with the patient, caregivers, nurse, and doctor to help the patient relearn lost skills. Ongoing support from the doctor means a lot to the patient and family.

Outside Hospital

Rehabilitation can be continued in an inpatient or outpatient center or in a skilled nursing facility (depending on the amount of therapy the patient can tolerate) and then continued at home. Improvement is not always steady. There can be plateaus when nothing happens for days and even weeks. However, rehabilitation efforts should continue. Because most insurance pays only while the patient is making progress, the patient and the caregivers become key figures in continuing this process. Improvement can continue in some patients several years after a stroke.

Rehabilitation of the Cancer Patient

Health professionals might not think of recommending rehabilitation when cancer is the diagnosis, but many cancer patients are living longer and some can benefit from rehabilitation. Patients with few or easily controlled symptoms can function well, lead a normal life, and return to work while treatment continues. They do not need rehabilitation. However, patients who have lost function can benefit. The more independent they can become, the better for their self-respect and the easier it makes life for their caregivers.

Self-care, mobility, and control of bowel and bladder are the functional giants. The rehabilitation team can design a program based on the severity of the cancer effects and define reasonable goals. The program can start in the hospital after operative or other treatment, or at an outpatient rehabilitation department, and continue at home with help from caregivers and friends. The rehabilitation team can be consulted as needed and in some cases may make home visits.

15

Community Resources

The array of resources available to assist elderly patients and their families is complex and fragmented. Not every resource is available in every community. A medical social worker should be able to give advice about local and national support systems, including the following examples.

LOCAL RESOURCES

- **Local hospitals** may offer a Social Service Department, volunteers, and publications about health, illness, and other resources.
- **Senior centers** and **community centers** may offer health education and screening, nutrition and outreach programs, and social and recreational activities. Some publish a yearly booklet of all the resources available in the community.
- **Agency on Aging** or **Local Council on Aging**. Most communities have some variation of these. They provide outreach programs and access to other resources such as senior centers, community centers, day care centers for patients with Alzheimer's dementia, and legal and financial aid.
- **Case management services**. Case management services can provide some frail elders and their

caregivers help coordinating the multiple factors which can affect their health and function. Case management can identify personal, social, and financial needs, and develop supportive services, thus helping the elder to stay independent in his or her home. Some are fee-for-service and can be expensive; some are subsidized by the community and are low-cost or no-cost. With all of these services, the small print must be read carefully before signing anything, and advice should be sought from the Social Service Department at the local hospital or from the area Agency on Aging.

- **Meals on Wheels** brings food to homebound elderly. The need is greater than the services available.
- The **Public Health Department** provides health information and referral services.
- **Hospice and Respite Care**. (See Part 6, At the End of Life.)

NATIONAL RESOURCES

- **Nationwide Societies**. Examples include the American Heart Association, American Cancer Society, and the Alzheimer's Association. The local hospital will have a list of such resources as well as educational literature from them, which is usually free. The American Cancer Society and local hospitals sponsor the "I Can Cope" program, one example of a helpful resource. Presentations about how cancer can affect health, finances, and legal affairs (wills, living wills, advance directives) are made to cancer patients and their caregivers by panels of experts including physicians, lawyers, nurses, and medical social workers. There is time for questions and discussion with other individuals in a similar situation.
- **American Association of Retired Persons (AARP)**. AARP is a large, growing group of Americans aged 50 and older, with significant power to lobby both state and federal government. Their glossy magazine, "Modern Maturity," is read by 30 million Americans every month. They produce

leaflets, booklets, tapes, and videos on every topic relating to aging, and conduct a reasonably priced mail-order medication service.

- The **American Society on Aging** has a wealth of information on aging, runs an educational Summer Series on Aging each year in five major cities, and organizes an annual meeting with sessions for both health professionals and lay people of all ages.

- **National Association of Area Agencies on Aging (NAAAA).** The NAAAA can provide contact information for agencies on aging for each state. The state agencies can provide information about adult protective services (or the equivalent) for a specific state. Their address is 927 15th Street, N.W., 6th Floor, Washington, D.C. 20005. They can also be reached by phone at (202) 296-8130, and by fax at (202) 296-8134.

- The **National Council on Aging** has many resources on aging and "constituent units" including:

  - National Institute of Senior Centers
  - National Adult Day Services Association
  - National Association of Older Worker Employment Services
  - National Center on Rural Aging
  - National Institute on Financial Issues and Services for Elders
  - National Institute of Senior Housing
  - Health Promotion Institute
  - National Institute on Community-based Long-term Care
  - National Interfaith Coalition on Aging

WHO PAYS FOR HEALTH CARE?

Medicare

Medicare is available to all Americans age 65 and older who are eligible for Social Security, as well as to those under age 65 who receive Social Security disability benefits after 2 years of permanent disability.

Medicare Part A covers inpatient hospital services and a limited amount of skilled nursing care.

Medicare Part B covers physician services and some additional services.

Medicaid

Medicaid helps to pay medical bills for individuals of any age with very low income. Eligibility varies from state to state. Medicaid is the major payor for long-term care in the United States. The nearest Social Security Office or Office of Social Services has details.

Continuation of Medicaid funding at the present level is a favorite topic of debate in the federal government. Cuts in welfare programs have already happened, harming the poorest, most vulnerable people in our society. Further budget cuts are likely and will bring with them an increase in malnutrition, neglect, and the diseases produced by poverty.

"Medigap" Policies

"Medigap" policies, available from commercial insurance companies, supplement Medicare benefits, and are paid for out-of-pocket by the senior. They range in price from hundreds to thousands of dollars a year. Because they are recent, their performance records are minimal. Some of them offer health benefits that are already covered under Medicare.

The National Association of Insurance Commissioners (NAIC) is collecting information about such policies. The local senior center or the Agency on Aging knows how to contact the NAIC and also has information about these policies.

Veterans Administration (VA)

In theory, VA health benefits are for veterans with service-connected disabilities and illnesses. However, because it can be difficult to decide whether an illness or adverse event that occurs years after serving in the armed forces is service connected, in practice VA health coverage is more generous than might be expected. A variety of health-care services may be covered at little or no cost to the veteran.

Several geriatric research and education centers, geriatric assessment units, and home health programs also have been developed by the VA.

Any person who has served at any time in any branch of the U.S. military should contact the nearest VA office for further details of what health benefits are available.

Health Insurance Plans and Managed Care for the Elderly

Seniors can assign their Medicare benefits to a commercial health insurance plan, which is then supposed to cover most of their health needs, in some cases including medications. Advise your patients to read the small print and ask many questions, especially about coverage for skilled nursing facility care, home care, and rehabilitation. Both "for profit" and "not for profit" plans have the objective of accumulating dollars to fund the plan and to pay administrative costs; often this is accomplished by manipulating deductibles, hidden costs, and exclusions.

"Managed-care" health plans for all ages of members currently include many different kinds of health insurance and health care plans. One of them is the Medicare HMO, in which the government reimburses the plan 95% of the average cost of caring for a senior on Medicare in its region, every month, for each enrollee. Healthy elderly people in states like Florida and California, with high populations of retirees, have been targeted by high-pressure salespersons working on commission for such plans. The plan salespersons try to recruit healthy elders who do not use expensive health resources. When seniors assign their Medicare benefits to one of these plans, they have to go to the doctors that the plan employs or contracts with, and so may have to give up their regular physician.

At best, the Medicare HMO works well, with no exclusions for previous or existing illness, no premiums, and no deductibles. The charge for each doctor visit is often less than $10. The best of these plans offer preventive health care such as health appraisals, eye examinations, dental care, and even exercise classes, and have programs to help the frail and sick elderly. They employ interdisciplinary health professional teams and case-manage as needed. A broad range of board-certified specialists is available, and the primary care doctors are either board certified or in the process of attaining this credential. They have at least one geriatrician on staff, and the HMO is involved in medical education and health research. The cost of medications may or may not be covered.

The worst Medicare HMOs exclude the sick elderly, limit access to care, and refuse coverage for necessary stays in nursing homes and rehabilitation after an acute illness, for instance. They may not have a full range of specialists on staff, and are unlikely to have a geriatrician available. They have little or no medical education or research interest. They may impose a dollar limit or a maximum lifetime benefit for certain expensive disorders, after which the enrollee is no longer covered. Doctors in the plan have to get permission, often from a nonmedical clerical person, before they can order needed tests or procedures. There are many shades of gray in Medicare HMOs between the best and the worst.

Although it is easy to disenroll from such a plan by filling in a disenrollment form at the local Social Security office or by notifying the plan in writing (use certified mail to have proof of delivery), a problem can arise. Medicare coverage begins on the first day of the month after notification of disenrollment. If an acute illness arises before reinstatement in Medicare, especially if in-hospital intensive care is needed, the senior's finances can quickly be wiped out.

Complaints (best in writing with relevant facts, times, and dates) can also be made about denial of services or other concerns. Initial complaints to the Medicare HMO itself might prove ineffective, however. (Quis custodiat custodies?) If this complaint does not produce results, an appeal to the state's Department of Corporations (DOC) would be next. (In most States, the DOC requires that a complaint be filed with the health plan first unless it is an emergency.) The Department of Health Services and the U.S. Health Care Financing Administration can also be contacted. Linking up with local consumer advocacy groups, the area Agency on Aging, the Gray Panthers, or AARP is also a good idea—they all have knowledge and experience and are ready and willing to share and help.

5
PART

Medications

16
CHAPTER

Prescribing for the Elderly: General Principles

The young physician starts life having 20 drugs for each disease and the old physician ends life by having one drug for 20 diseases.
Sir William Osler (1849–1919)

If we would throw into the sea all the drugs we know, it would be so much the better for the patients, and so much the worse for the fishes!
Oliver Wendell Holmes (1809–1894)

What a distrust of medications is expressed in these quotations! The words of Osler and Holmes, both distinguished physicians and thoughtful men, acknowledge the potential for damage inherent in drugs. They also reveal reservations about the judgment of members of their own profession!

CAUSES OF
MEDICATION-RELATED PROBLEMS

We know that every medication has both good and bad effects, and that the elderly are particularly vulnerable to the bad ones. More than 25% of all medications in the United States today are consumed by persons 65 or older, and on average this group uses four or more medications, often simultaneously. In the same group, 15% to 20% of admissions to acute-care hospitals are related to medication reactions, and death from them is not unknown.

Several factors contribute to the high medication consumption in this group: multiple pathology, multiple physicians and caregivers, inadequate clinical assessment, influence of friends and family, drug company advertising, and unrealistic expectations of both patient and doctor—the "pill for every ill" and the "perhaps death is optional" attitudes. (See Chap. 17 for further discussion of these factors.)

Physiological aging itself increases medication-related problems because of:

- Reduced homeostatic responses in the elderly
- Reduced number of some medication receptor target organs in the tissues
- Changes in target-organ sensitivity
- Increased body fat: fat-soluble medications are recycled and stored longer
- Decreased serum albumin in many frail elderly

PRINCIPLES OF PRESCRIBING FOR
THE ELDERLY: TAKE CARE!

The most important things to remember about prescribing for the elderly can be summarized by a most appropriate acronym: CARE.

C is for "Caution"

- Prescribe cautiously. Consider *risk* versus *benefit* for the proposed therapy.

- Is the medication really necessary? Will the disorder resolve without medication?
- Is there an effective nonmedication option, such as physical or occupational therapy, counseling, biofeedback, exercise, or a change in diet or lifestyle?
- Prescribe for a specific indication and stop the drug if it is no longer needed.
- Will the drug being considered compromise the patient's function?
- KISS! (Keep it simple, sweetie!) Keep the list of drugs as short as possible. Do not attempt to medicate every problem on the patient's list. You will poison him or her if you do that.
- Consider the patient's renal and hepatic function and the effect on drug detoxification.

C is for "Compliance"

- Prescribe a liquid format if the patient has difficulty swallowing pills. If no liquid format is available, consider crushing the medication and mixing it with applesauce. (This is not a good idea with sustained-release or enteric-coated preparations.)
- The pharmacist can substitute nonchildproof caps. These can be essential for patients with arthritis in their hands or wrists. Some pharmacists require the patient to sign a waiver of responsibility.
- How good is the patient's memory? Can he or she follow the drug schedule?
- How good is the patient's vision? Clear labeling is essential, with large print if necessary.
- How expensive is the medication? Consider the state of the patient's finances.
- Will the dosage scheme make compliance easy? Most patients can manage twice daily (BID), but few stay with four times daily (QID).

A is for "Adjust Dosage with Age"

- Start *low*, go *slow*. (Antibiotics and insulin can be exceptions.) Large loading doses are usually

unnecessary. Use a limited number of drugs and know them well. Every-other-day (QOD) dosage can work for medications with a long half-life, but may be more difficult for the patient to remember.
- Because body fat increases with age, adjust the dosage of fat-soluble medications.
- Lower serum albumin can affect action of protein-bound drugs.

R is for "Review Regimen Regularly"

- Can any medications be discontinued? Does the need for them still exist? Would episodic treatment with fewer side effects be as effective as a continuous course?
- Distinguish between a new symptom and a side effect of a previously prescribed drug. Avoid the common error of treating an undesirable medication effect with another medication. The only time this is justified is in hospice (see Part 6) or if there is no alternative to the prescribed drug, and the benefit is real.
- Avoid automatic refills for prolonged periods.
- Maintain a high index of suspicion for drug-induced adverse effects, which can produce almost any symptom in any organ system. They may present as nonspecific symptoms of lethargy or malaise (see "Failure to Thrive" in Chap. 8), or as a decrease in the patient's ability to perform basic activities of daily living (ADLs) or instrumental activities of daily living (IADLs). Confusion, depression, dizziness, syncopal episodes, and falls can all be caused by drugs.
- Look for other sources of medication. Patients sometimes obtain drugs from family members or friends. They may also consult with other physicians or buy over-the-counter or alternative medicine and herbal remedies. Patients can fill in a medication checklist at home or while waiting to see you in the office. (See Appendix C for one example.) This checklist can be filed in their chart and updated at each subsequent visit.

E is for "Educate"

- Present drug information via leaflets, newsletters, or handouts. Many of these are available free or at low cost from community, hospital, or pharmacy medication education programs.
- Use the expertise of local pharmacists to counsel your patients and do mini drug reviews.
- Make sure your patients know the name of each drug prescribed for them, what it is for, and the major side effects. The caveat here is that studies show that patients of any age who are told about drug side effects display more of them.
- Emphasize *when* the drug is likely to start producing its beneficial effects so that a disappointed patient will not stop therapy prematurely.
- A wallet medication card that is kept current can be valuable for both the patient and the physician.

17
CHAPTER

How Do Problems with Medications Occur?

PROBLEMS WITH PRESCRIBING PRACTICES OR COMPLIANCE

- **Overprescribing or inappropriate prescribing.** Studies show that the older the patient, the more likely the doctor is to prescribe a medication. The quick fix can be tempting—to write a prescription instead of taking the *time* needed to listen to the patient and do a risk-benefit analysis on the multiple problems presented. (As noted in earlier chapters, an attempt to medicate every problem will poison the patient.) Also, many patients are not satisfied unless they are given a prescription. The "exchange of gifts" idea, in which the doctor always feels obliged to give the patient something more tangible than medical judgment, is treacherous. Some patients, brainwashed by advertising that says "Ask your doctor about. . .," put pressure on the doctor to give them a medication. When you add to this the constant pressure on doctors from pharmaceutical companies to prescribe their products, it is hardly surprising that overprescribing to the elderly is a major, sometimes deadly, problem. (Remember, 15% to 20% of hospital admissions in the over-65 age group are linked with medication side effects.) **PEARL: Instead of falling into the prescription trap, *think function!* How will the medication affect it?**

- **Lack of review and coordination of all medications** every 6 to 12 months by the patient's health professional.
- **Schedule too complicated** to follow easily: this usually means too many medicines, more room for error, and trouble. Keep it simple!
- **Self-medication by the patient** with drugs saved from previous therapy or borrowed from a friend.
- **Self-medication by the patient** with drugs bought without a prescription at the pharmacy. Ask patients to take a list of all their medications to the pharmacy when buying any nonprescription drug. The pharmacist can check for adverse interactions.
- **Noncompliance with instructions**. Video studies have shown that many doctors either lack communication skills or do not take the time required to make instructions clear to patients. Even if the doctor explains instructions well, many patients (at every age) remember only a small fraction of what was said to them at the office visit.

  1. **Underuse or omission** is the most common problem and could be caused by any or all of the following factors:

     - Simple forgetting, especially when the patient starts to feel better
     - Poor memory or confusion
     - Inability to buy medication because of high cost of drugs
     - A lack of understanding of how important it is to *complete* the course of the medicine
     - Depression with reduced motivation
     - Not getting expected results soon enough

     PEARL: The use of a plastic container with a medication compartment for each day of the month can overcome some of the problems of medication underuse or omission. It can be filled with all current medications once a month by the patient, a caregiver, nurse, or pharmacist. It also makes it easier to check whether medications have been taken. I have seen patients with significant memory loss use this system with only minimal help.

2. **Overuse, erratic use, and contraindicated use**, either deliberate or accidental, can all lead to problems. Advise the patient not to keep medicine bottles at the bedside. The wrong drug, a wrong dose, or a second dose could be taken in the middle of the night. If a dose is needed in the dark, make sure that only the exact amount is by the bedside and no more. Do not put different pills together in one bottle.

- **Use of time-expired medicines**. Some become toxic with time and others become ineffective.
- **Not being able to get the cap off the bottle**.

WHICH ELDERLY ARE MOST AT RISK FOR MEDICATION PROBLEMS?

- Those who are isolated
- "Doctor shoppers" who end up with multiple providers and uncoordinated multiple medications
- Those with poor memory or mental confusion
- Those who are depressed: they lack the motivation to bother about their plan of treatment
- People with poor vision
- Patients with arthritis
- Alcoholic patients
- Poor patients: if they have no insurance and cannot afford a medication, they do without
- Patients who don't speak the same language as the doctor and have no one to translate for them
- People recovering from recent serious illness or hospital stay
- Patients with unrealistic expectations who demand instant cure
- Bored and discontented people who expect a drug to change their life

WHICH MEDICATIONS ARE MOST OFTEN ASSOCIATED WITH PROBLEMS?

Nonprescription Medications

The most frequently consumed nonprescription drugs are antacids, analgesics, vitamins and minerals, laxatives, cold remedies, and cough syrups. Several of these groups are commonly associated with problems.

Aspirin (ASA) and Preparations Containing It

Stomach irritation and bleeding are common. The older and frailer the patient, the less well he or she tolerates blood loss, which can result in anemia or dizziness. These preparations also can interact with anticoagulants.

Loss of high-frequency hearing can be the first sign of aspirin (ASA) overdose in the elderly. Because this occurs with normal aging, distinguishing between normal and abnormal hearing loss can be difficult. Tinnitus, which is an early warning of toxicity in younger age groups, often does not occur in older people.

Nonsteroidal Anti-inflammatory Drugs (NSAIDs)

NSAIDs are useful medications, but they can cause any of the following problems in the elderly:

- Stomach irritation
- Bleeding
- Gastroesophageal reflux disease
- Peptic ulcer disease
- Chronic constipation
- Fluid retention, which can worsen hypertension and congestive heart failure
- Lessened effectiveness of some antihypertensive medications

- Depression in some patients
- Impaired coordination, with a higher incidence of falls

Antihistamines

The antihistamines found in cough, cold, and allergy remedies can cause:

- Hypertension
- Confusion
- Constipation
- Urinary retention
- Blurring of vision
- Exacerbation of glaucoma
- Reduced effectiveness of other drugs

Laxatives

Inappropriate laxative use can cause electrolyte imbalance, dehydration, or reduced effectiveness of other medications as a result of intestinal hurry.

Antacids

Many antacids are high in sodium. Also, they can interfere with the effects of other medications, render tetracyclines ineffective, and cause diarrhea.

Prescription Medications

Some medications have paradoxical effects. For example, a tranquilizer may cause excitement and agitation instead of calming; a sleeping pill may cause insomnia.

Digoxin

Digoxin can cause anorexia, nausea, vomiting, cardiac arrhythmias, or mental confusion.

Diuretics

The use of diuretics can lead to dehydration, hypokalemia, confusion, weakness, postural hypotension, and falls.

Anticoagulants

Beware of drug interactions and bleeding. A recent study has shown that the anticlotting effect of anticoagulants can be increased by acetaminophen, one of the most commonly consumed medications, either alone or in combination. Some elders taking low doses of anticoagulants prophylactically (e.g., after total joint replacement) may be at risk for drug interactions; many surgeons are switching to ASA because of the risks of anticoagulants. (See Chap. 19.)

Sedatives

Sedatives can produce confusion, a hungover feeling the next day, rebound insomnia, or worsening of sleep apnea. Sedatives combined with alcohol can be deadly.

ASA and NSAIDs

Prescription versions of these drugs, which generally have a higher dose in each pill, cause the same problems as the nonprescription forms. The level of drug in the body can be similar for both forms, depending on how many pills are taken.

18
CHAPTER

Prescribing for Some Common Disorders

Common disorders occur commonly in every age group, so you will spend much of your medical practice prescribing and managing medications for the following conditions: hypertension, glaucoma, diabetes mellitus, thyroid disease, degenerative joint disease, and arthralgia. This chapter points out some special caveats to be observed when dealing with elderly patients with these disorders. (The American Society of Geriatrics current standards of practice for anticoagulation in the elderly follow in Chap. 19.)

HYPERTENSION

In western societies, blood pressure usually rises with age, secondary to increased peripheral resistance. This means that intra-arterial pressures can be lower than sphygmomanometer readings and antihypertensive drugs must be prescribed with caution, especially for the very elderly. Decreased brain perfusion can lead to confusion, dizziness, and falls. Decreased perfusion of extremities can lead to skin breakdown. If the patient is being treated for chronic glaucoma (discussed later), proceed with caution and consult with the ophthalmologist.

Isolated systolic hypertension is found in about 20% of seniors and must be managed with caution; dropping the normal diastolic pressure too low can damage the patient.

Although hypertension statistically increases morbidity and mortality, particularly from myocardial infarction and stroke, clinical judgment must still be applied to each patient and the side effects of treatment, especially injury and loss of function, weighed against possible benefits.

In most cases, nondrug treatment can be tried first:

- Decreased sodium intake
- Weight loss
- Gentle exercise
- **No tobacco**
- Reduced alcohol consumption or no alcohol
- Stress management
- Pain control

If medication is needed, there are many factors to consider. Renal and hepatic function and plasma volume may be decreased. The presence of other chronic diseases such as diabetes mellitus also should influence choice of drug. Polypharmacy produces side effects and unfavorable drug interactions. And remember that the cost of medication can affect compliance.

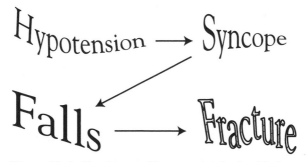

Figure 18-1. The danger of hypotension in the elderly.

Table 18–1. COMPARISON OF COMMONLY PRESCRIBED MEDICATIONS FOR HYPERTENSION

Type of Medication	Cost	Advantages	Problems
Diuretics	Low	Useful in CHF, COPD Decreased incidence of hip fracture with thiazides Best used in low doses	Syncope, dehydration, hypokalemia, hyperglycemia, hyperuricemia, impotence, ototoxicity (with loop diuretics), photosensitivity
Beta blockers	Moderate	Can use in IHD, some arrhythmias, CHF with diastolic dysfunction, migraine, gout Can give long-acting preparation QD, HS	Less effective in elderly Can cause bradycardia, heart block, syncope, impotence, depression, confusion Don't use in COPD, asthma, heart block, PVD, DM
Alpha blockers	Moderate	Can use in CHF, COPD, asthma, gout, BPH, DM, renal impairment, PVD	Syncope, dizziness, fluid retention, dry mouth, urinary incontinence

Calcium channel blockers	Moderate to high	Can use in IHD, COPD, DM, PVD, gout Use with caution in CHF	Syncope, heart block, reflex tachycardia, bradycardia Can cause CHF, constipation, urinary retention, edema
ACE inhibitors	Moderate to high	Can use in CHF, DM, gout, PVD	Syncope, hyperkalemia, azotemia, chronic cough NSAIDs may make less effective

BPH = benign prostatic hypertrophy, CHF = congestive heart failure, COPD = chronic obstructive pulmonary disease, DM = diabetes mellitus, IHD = ischemic heart disease, PVD = peripheral vascular disease.

Tailor the drug regimen to the individual patient, weighing risks versus benefits (Table 18–1). **PEARL: Consider how antihypertensive drug treatment will affect the patient's functioning. In general, start with a low dose and go slow with hypertension medications.** Side effects such as hypotension can have unwelcome consequences (Fig. 18–1). *Keep the regimen as simple as possible!*

GLAUCOMA

The primary care practitioner and the ophthalmologist should each be aware of the medications the other is prescribing. Many glaucoma medications produce adverse side effects in elderly patients:

- **Topical medications**
  - **Miotics** (pilocarpine, carbachol): headache, nausea, bronchospasm
  - **Adrenergics** (epinephrine): eye irritation, allergic lid reaction, hypertension, tachycardia, headache
  - **Beta blockers**: bradycardia, congestive heart failure, bronchospasm
- **Systemic medications**
  - **Carbonic anhydrase inhibitors** (acetazolamide): anorexia, nausea, fatigue, paresthesias, confusion, systemic acidosis, renal stones, skin rashes, bone marrow suppression

Conversely, some medications frequently prescribed for other disorders can make glaucoma worse:

- **Antihypertensive medications**: Optic nerve nutrition depends on a balance between intraocular pressure (IOP) and blood pressure (BP). If BP is being lowered, IOP may need to be reduced more to maintain optic nerve nutrition.
- **Anticholinergics**: These can cause pupillary dilatation, leading to angle closure glaucoma. They also can antagonize anti-glaucoma medication.

DIABETES MELLITUS (DM)

Epidemiology

Diabetes mellitus comes in two types: insulin-dependent (type I, IDDM) and non–insulin-dependent (type II, NIDDM). After age 45, 98% of all DM is NIDDM. Among those between ages 65 and 75, 18% suffer from it, as do 40% of those over 80.

Native Americans have the highest incidence of DM in the world. Hispanics are three times more likely to develop DM than non-Hispanics, and Hispanics with NIDDM are six times more likely to develop renal disease requiring dialysis, and two to three times more likely to develop retinopathy than non-Hispanics.

Asians in the United States have a higher incidence of NIDDM than comparable groups in their native lands.

African Americans over age 65 are three times more likely to develop DM than whites, and DM is the third leading cause of death in African Americans.

Clinical Presentation

DM can present in the elderly as failure to thrive, with fatigue and lethargy, or with a complication such as a foot ulcer, peripheral neuropathy, poor vision, or renal failure (Fig. 18–2).

Slowly developing mental confusion in the elderly diabetic is most commonly caused by hypoglycemia; hyperglycemic pre-coma or coma, which may be hyperosmolar (more common in the elderly diabetic) or ketotic; cerebrovascular accident; silent myocardial infarction; or infection.

Insulin resistance can develop with aging. It can cause glucose intolerance, dyslipidemia, or hypertension with increased risk of coronary artery disease (CAD).

Management of the Elderly Diabetic

The general principles of management are the same as for younger age groups, but the elderly in general

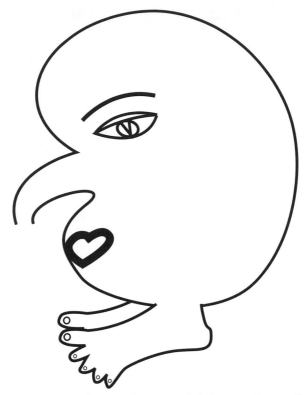

Figure 18–2. The complications of diabetes mellitus. All systems are disordered, but the organs most affected are the kidneys, eyes, cardiovascular system, and feet.

are at higher risk for hypoglycemia (which kills brain cells) and impaired renal and hepatic function. They may also have multiple pathology and medications. **PEARL: Frail elderly diabetics, either at home or in a skilled nursing facility (SNF), do better overall with less rigid control of blood glucose.** A degree of hyperglycemia harms them less than episodes of hypoglycemia and allows a more liberal diet.

Realistic and *achievable* goals for each individual elderly patient with diabetes must be defined. A good mnemonic for management of the diabetic is **DEEM:**

Diet
Exercise
Education
Medications

Diet

The first step for all diabetics is to control total calorie intake, of which 10% to 20% should be from protein, less than 30% from fat, and the rest from complex carbohydrates. Intake should include enough fiber, moderate sodium, no alcohol or a moderate amount, a multivitamin with minerals, vitamin C (500 mg), and vitamin E (400 IU).

Control of calorie intake is important even if the patient is taking antidiabetic medications as directed. An uncontrolled diet can result in hyperglycemia, which causes visual disturbances, increased risk of infection, cardiovascular problems, and polyuria, which can lead to dehydration and electrolyte imbalance.

Risk factors for poor nutrition in the elderly fit the mnemonic **AID:**

A   Anorexia, leading to hypoglycemia
    Arthritis, hindering the preparation of food
I   Immobility (can't get to store or to cooking appliances)
    Income limited
    Impaired cognition
    Impaired caregiver
D   Dental problems or dentures not fitting
    Depression

Exercise

Exercise is good for everyone, not just diabetics. Any form of exercise that the patient enjoys and is likely to pursue will produce the following benefits: weight loss (maybe); improved circulation, appetite, and sleep; normalization of glucose (increased uptake into muscle cells); increased number of insulin receptors; and improvement in depression. Commitment to regular meetings, such as walking groups or an exercise class, provides social contacts and makes it more likely that the patient will continue.

Education

The management of DM is complex. In educating the patient, caregiver, or both, you first will need to determine their first language and whether they are literate. Also assess special senses and mental state.

Aspects to be taught include:

- Monitoring of blood glucose by the patient or caregiver.
- The symptoms, signs, and treatment of hypoglycemia.
- Adjustments to be made in treatment if the patient is sick.
- Importance of regular foot inspection and care by a nurse or podiatrist.
- Importance of regular eye checks.
- Psychosocial issues: impact on patient and caregivers of a long-term, complex disorder. Support groups are helpful.
- Interaction with other medications. Advise the patient to check with his or her physician before adding any new prescription or nonprescription medication or alternative therapy.

The American Diabetes Association has helpful programs and leaflets for patients and caregivers.

Medications

If diet and exercise have not worked, drug therapy is next.

How to Choose?

Factors to consider in choosing a regimen of medications for an elderly patient with DM include:

- How obese is the patient?
- What co-morbid conditions does the patient have?
- How good is renal and hepatic function?

- What medications is the patient currently taking—prescription, nonprescription, and alternative therapies?
- What is the blood glucose level after fasting all night and 1 hour after the main meal?
- What is the result of the C-peptide blood test? (gives insulin profile.)
- What is the glycated (glycosylated) hemoglobin (HbA1c) blood level? (This gives the average blood glucose concentration over the last 2 to 3 months; it might not reveal shorter-term peaks and troughs.)
- How compliant is the patient or caregiver likely to be?
- What is the cost to the patient of the proposed regimen?

Oral Monotherapy

Sulfonylureas

The second-generation sulfonylureas (such as glyburide, glipizide, glimepiride) are preferable to the first-generation preparations (such as tolbutamide) because they have shorter half lives, fewer interactions with other drugs, and fewer side effects. Start with half the dose used for younger patients and titrate up slowly.

This group of medications increases the release of insulin from the pancreas, increases insulin receptors, and reduces hepatic glucose production. They are contraindicated for patients with severe hepatic or renal insufficiency.

Biguanides (Metformin)

Metformin enhances insulin-stimulated glucose transport in skeletal muscle and decreases hepatic glucose production. It does not cause hypoglycemia and has favorable effects on blood lipids—it lowers total cholesterol, lowers triglycerides, and lowers LDL cholesterol (the "bad" kind for the cardiovascular system). Metformin is synergistic with sulphonylureas.

A possible side effect is lactic acidosis, characterized by malaise, myalgias, respiratory distress, low blood pH, and elevated plasma lactate. This rare but deadly effect is more likely to occur in hepatic or renal dysfunction.

In elderly patients, start low (500 mg twice daily [BID] with food) and take at least 6 weeks to reach the maximum dose (2000 mg daily in divided doses). Metformin has a good effect on clotting factors. It can cause a decrease in B_{12} and folate, which should be measured in the first few months of therapy.

Contraindications include decreased renal function, risk of sepsis or cardiovascular decompensation, or alcoholism or binge drinking. Also, it should not be used in persons receiving IV contrast agents or those with a rapidly deteriorating medical condition.

Alpha-Glucosidase Inhibitors (acarbose)

These drugs block the absorption of complex carbohydrates, but have no effect on glucose or lactate. They can be used with diet, insulin, or other oral agents, and can be given at mealtimes. The main side effect is flatulence. Build up the dose gradually, starting with 25 mg three times daily (TID) with the first bite of each meal. Increase to 100 mg TID. They do not cause hypoglycemia and have a stool-softening effect.

These drugs have been used successfully with insulin to decrease the insulin dose and give smoother control. They inhibit hepatic glucose output, decrease intestinal glucose absorption, and facilitate weight loss.

Troglitazone (Rezulin)

This drug improves the insulin response of peripheral target tissue, increasing glucose metabolism and tolerance and decreasing insulin concentrations. It works well in elderly patients with insulin resistance and has minimal side effects. It can expand blood volume, however, which could precipitate or worsen congestive heart failure (CHF).

Oral Combination Therapy

Any of these oral monotherapeutic agents can be combined if the monotherapy regimen fails. (See Table 18–2.) Start low, go slow.

Table 18–2. HOW TO MANAGE FAILURES OF ORAL THERAPY FOR DIABETES MELLITUS

Failed Regimen	Sulfonylureas	Metformin	Sulfonylureas and Metformin	Sulfonylurea, Metformin, and Acarbose
Overall poor control	Add metformin	Add sulfonylurea, then acarbose	Switch to insulin	Switch to insulin
Fasting hyperglycemia	Add HS isophane (NPH) insulin	Add HS isophane (NPH) insulin	Add HS isophane (NPH) insulin	Add HS isophane (NPH) insulin
Postprandial hyperglycemia	Add acarbose or lispro insulin	Add acarbose or lispro insulin	Add acarbose or lispro insulin	Add lispro insulin
Other	Poor control with low C-peptide: needs insulin		Borderline poor control: add acarbose	Obese NIDDM: reduce weight, consider anorexics. Lean NIDDM or low C-peptide: needs insulin

Insulin

Apply the same guidelines as for younger patients, but remember that the elderly are more susceptible to hypoglycemia, and, because of mental or physical disability, they may be less able to administer insulin and monitor its effects.

Lispro insulin (brand name Humalog) is a recently developed human insulin analog that is faster acting than regular insulin and has a shorter duration of action. It can be useful for some diabetics because it allows more flexible dosing. As with the management of all insulin-dependent diabetics of any age, the patient's total lifestyle, weight, diet, general health, and individual metabolic needs must be considered.

Acarbose has been used successfully in combination with insulin for many years in other countries to improve weight control and fasting and postprandial blood glucose, and to prevent hypoglycemia.

Aspirin (ASA)

If there are no contraindications such as renal or liver failure, a history of gastrointestinal (GI) bleeding, or a likelihood of drug interactions, most clinicians recommend that diabetics take an aspirin daily, with food, for the favorable cardiovascular effects. For most diabetics, 80 to 160 mg daily (1–2 baby aspirins) is enough. If there is a history of heart attack or stroke, up to 325 mg can be taken daily.

THYROID DISEASE

Thyroid disease most often presents atypically and insidiously in the elderly and can be difficult to diagnose clinically. Failure to thrive, falling, constipation, confusion, and even (in rare cases) delirium (myxedema madness) can be presenting features. Cardiovascular effects, such as heart failure and atrial fibrillation (AF), are seen in many cases. **PEARL: Keep a high index of suspicion for thyroid disease in your elderly patients.** Thyroid function studies, including sensitive TSH, usually make the diagnosis clear and allow prompt initiation of treatment.

Hypothyroidism

The treatment for hypothyroidism is L-thyroxine. The average daily dose for patients over age 65 is 0.075 to 0.1 mg. Start with 0.025 mg daily and increase by 0.025-mg increments at intervals of at least 2 weeks. In the patient with ischemic heart disease, start with 0.0125 mg per day, and use smaller incremental doses.

Two months after reaching 0.075 mg per day, measure TSH. If it is greater than normal, increase the dose to 0.1 mg. If it is lower than normal, lower the dose. Because serum TSH can fall slowly, if the TSH is still high 2 months after a dose of 0.1 mg per day is reached, wait another 2 months before increasing the dose to 0.125 mg per day.

Watch for cardiac arrhythmias, angina, or dyspnea during treatment.

Hyperthyroidism

This condition is treated with radioactive iodine (^{131}I), antithyroid medications, or β-blockers (which do not inhibit thyroid function, but temporarily suppress signs and symptoms).

About two-thirds of hyperthyroid elderly patients with AF revert *spontaneously* in the first 4 months after becoming euthyroid. Psychiatric symptoms caused by the thyroid disease also usually clear after the patient becomes euthyroid.

DEGENERATIVE JOINT DISEASE (DJD)

Medication and Other Nonsurgical Management

- **Pain control. PEARL: Treating joint pain lets the joints move more freely. This maintains muscle strength, which in turn protects the afflicted joints.**

  - In established DJD, inflammation is not a major feature. ASA and NSAIDs (nonsteroidal anti-inflammatory drugs), with their significant side effects, are contraindicated in the management of the pain. Acetaminophen (Tylenol), Tylenol with codeine, or Vicodin are safer medications to prescribe long-term. When using codeine-containing medications or codeine analogues such as Vicodin, prescribe a bowel regimen prophylactically; these medications all cause constipation in the elderly. (See the section on management of constipation in Chap. 8.)

- Occasional intra-articular injection of corticosteroids and local anesthetic can help. Frequent injection will produce steroid arthropathy.

- **Weight loss.** Though desirable, significant weight loss probably is not a realistic expectation for obese elderly patients. Those who have been obese all their lives are unlikely to change now.
- **Heat, cold, massage** of the affected joint, hydrotherapy
- **Daily exercise** to put joints through as full a range of motion as possible, and to strengthen muscles
- **Rest**, but not too much
- **Attention to posture** (poor posture makes arthritis worse)
- **Good nutrition**
- **Stress management**
- **Use of community resources** such as the Arthritis Foundation

Surgery

- **Arthrodesis:** gives a stable, stiff, pain-free joint
- **Joint replacement:** Replacement of hip and knee joints is particularly successful. It restores function and allows the patient to be mobilized almost immediately. The pain-free patient can move more easily, decreasing demands on the heart (helpful in patients with a fragile cardiovascular system).

- **Osteotomy:** An alternative to joint replacement, more often used in younger patients or where no good prosthesis is available.

ARTHRALGIA

Aging can bring with it a collection of minor aches and pains. If a history and physical, complete blood count (CBC), sedimentation rate, and uric acid are all within normal limits, the most important considerations are:

- What causes the pains? Can these factors be modified?
- What helps the pains?
- Do the pains compromise the patient's function?
- Is the patient depressed? Constant chronic pain may be producing a reactive depression, or the pains could be a symptom of masked depression.

These minor aches and pains may be helped by measures such as the following:

- As much **exercise** as the patient can tolerate. Swimming is excellent exercise and easy on aching joints. Yoga and tai chi both emphasize controlled flexibility and can improve posture, muscle strength, and sleep.
- **Avoiding isolation**. The patient should get involved! Suggest that he or she join a walking group for exercise and company. Mall walking has become popular in areas of the country with extreme climates.
- **Weight loss if the patient is obese** is probably not realistic. People who have been this way all their lives are unlikely to change now.
- **Splints, wraps, heat, cold, rubs** such as Ben-Gay, Fire and Ice, etc. Ointment with ASA added can help some patients while avoiding the undesirable effects of oral ASA. Some elderly patients swear by capsaicin ointment.

- **Oral medications.** Start with plain Tylenol, or Tylenol with codeine. Salsalate is a low-toxicity preparation that can give relief. Low-toxicity NSAIDs may help.

PEARL: EVALUATION FOLLOWED BY REASSURANCE FROM THE PRACTITIONER THAT THERE IS NOTHING SERIOUSLY WRONG IS SOMETIMES ENOUGH TO RELIEVE ANXIETY AND MAKE THE ACHES AND PAINS TOLERABLE.

19

CHAPTER

Oral Anticoagulation Therapy for Older Adults

Great care must be taken when prescribing oral anticoagulants for any patient, but especially for the elderly. Nevertheless, there are several important indications for anticoagulation in the elderly:

- **Stroke prevention**. Long-term anticoagulation with oral warfarin is indicated for elderly patients with chronic atrial fibrillation (AF) unless they have a previous history of bleeding disorder, are at high risk for falls, have uncontrolled hypertension, or are taking essential medications that interact with warfarin. The risk of embolic stroke is increased in chronic AF, whether it is associated with valvular heart disease, cardiomyopathy, recent anterior wall myocardial infarction, hypertension, left ventricular hypertrophy, or previous transient ischemic attack (TIA).
- **Deep vein thrombosis**, with or without pulmonary embolism.

Table 19–1. ORAL ANTICOAGULANT GUIDELINES FOR PRACTICE*

Thromboembolic Disorder	INR	Duration	Clinical Comments
Venous Thromboembolism			
Prophylaxis (high-risk surgery)	2.0–3.0	≤3 months or until ambulatory	Alternatives include low molecular weight heparin or adjusted dose heparin. For hip replacement or major knee surgery, low molecular weight heparin begun 12 hours postoperative is more effective.
Treatment: Single episode (DVT or PE)	2.0–3.0	3–6 months	At or above the knee.
Treatment: Recurrent episode (DVT or PE)	2.0–3.0	3–6 months	Recurrent DVT or PE may require anticoagulation indefinitely.
Prevention of Systemic Embolism			
Atrial fibrillation (AF)	2.0–3.0	Indefinite	Warfarin, unless contraindicated; then consider ASA (325 mg/d).
AF: Cardioversion	2.0–3.0	3 weeks prior; 4 weeks post sinus rhythm	Consider indefinite anticoagulation in patients who do not cardiovert.

Condition	INR	Duration	Comments
Acute myocardial infarction	2.0–3.0	≤3 months	Patients with severe LV dysfunction, CHF, previous emboli, or 2-D echocardiographic evidence of mural thrombosis; indefinitely in patients with AF.[†] Indefinitely for secondary prevention of myocardial infarction in postinfarction patients unable to take daily ASA.[†]
Cardiomyopathy	2.0–3.0	Indefinite	Consider patient with ejection fraction ≤25% and high risk of SE.
Recurrent systemic embolism	2.0–3.0	Indefinite	Criteria for "recurrence": events, temporal and etiologic relationships.
Tissue heart valves	2.0–3.0	3 months	Followed by ASA (325 mg/d) indefinitely (optional).
Valvular heart disease	2.0–3.0	Indefinite	Consider only patients with a history of SE, AF, or left atrial diameter >5.5 cm. If recurrent embolism occurs, add ASA (80 mg/d) and/or increase INR to 2.5–3.5.
Mechanical prosthetic valves	2.5–3.5	Indefinite	If recurrent embolism occurs, add ASA (80 mg/d) or dipyridamole (400 mg/d). If high bleeding risk, INR 2.0–3.0 with or without ASA (80 mg/d).

INR = international normalized ratio; DVT = deep vein thrombosis; PE = pulmonary embolism; AF = atrial fibrillation; SE = systemic embolism; LV = left ventricular; CHF = congestive heart failure; ASA = aspirin.
*Modified from Chest 1995, 108:231S-470S and West J Med 1989, 151:414–429.
[†]Circulation 1996, 94:2341–2350.

Table 19–2. INITIATION OF ORAL ANTICOAGULATION WITH WARFARIN

Dosing Approach	Warfarin Dose		
	Day 1	Day 2	Day 3
Urgent	5–7.5 mg	5–7.5 mg	2–7.5 mg
Nonurgent	2–5 mg	2–5 mg	2–5 mg

Monitoring the Initiation of Oral Anticoagulation:

1. Nonurgent dosing can be used for chronic stable AF, for example, or if there is a bleeding risk.
2. Day 1 obtain baseline INR and therapeutic APTT (can be initiated with heparin on day 1).
3. Check INR daily until stable/therapeutic (usually 4–5 days), then 2–3 times a week for 2 weeks, weekly for one month, then monthly.
4. Warfarin dosing as Coumadin, available as 1, 2, 2.5, 3, 4, 5, 6, 7.5, and 10 mg tablets.

INR = international normalized ratio; AF = atrial fibrillation; APTT = activated partial thromboplastin time.

Table 19–3. REVERSAL OF ORAL ANTICOAGULANT EFFECT: NONBLEEDING

INR	Vitamin K Dose[†]	Route	Comments
6–10*	0.5–1.0 mg	PO, SC	PO absorption may be unpredictable in the elderly.
10–20	3.0–5.0 mg	SC, IV	Check INR in 6–12 h; repeat if necessary.
> 20	5.0–10.0 mg	SC, IV	Check INR in 6–12 h; repeat if necessary.

INR = international normalized ratio.
*Withholding warfarin may be considered.
[†]IV route may produce anaphylactic reaction; only Aqua Mephyton may be given IV.

- **Prosthetic heart valves**, either tissue or mechanical.
- **Acute myocardial infarction** with risk of mural thrombosis and systemic embolism.

Generally, however, the older the patient, the more fragile, and any blood loss, even small, may be poorly tolerated. The drop in blood pressure that blood loss can produce in the arteriosclerotic patient can lead to a heart attack or a stroke. The medical history of the patient must be reviewed for any bleeding tendencies, peptic ulcer disease, uncontrolled hypertension, falling, inability to comply with medications (e.g., in Alzheimer's dementia), or inability to comply with the frequent monitoring that will be needed. All of these would be contraindications to this form of therapy. *All medications*, including prescription, non-prescription, herbal, and alternative therapies, must be reviewed in detail and their interaction with the anticoagulants considered. **PEARL: The patient taking anticoagulants must be warned not to start new medication of any kind without consulting a doctor or a pharmacist.**

Table 19–4. REVERSAL OF ORAL ANTICOAGULANT EFFECT: BLEEDING

Extent of Bleeding	Warfarin Dose	Vitamin K*	FFP
Minor	Reduce	1 mg (PO, SC) if INR > 4.5 or withhold warfarin	—
Severe	Stop	5 mg SC, IV	Consider
Life-threatening	Stop	10 mg IV	Yes

FFP = fresh frozen plasma; INR = international normalized ratio.
*IV route may produce anaphylactic reaction; only Aqua Mephyton may be given IV.

The practice guidelines in Tables 19–1 through 19–4 were developed by the American Geriatrics Society* for managing different aspects of oral anticoagulation in the elderly, and are ideal for quick, easy reference. Practical guidance is given in Table 19–1 about when to use anticoagulation, the desirable international normalized ratio (INR) range in each situation, duration of therapy, and helpful clinical comments. Table 19–2 gives details on how to start treatment with warfarin, and Tables 19–3 and 19–4 show how to manage problems with anticoagulation, such as INR that is too high without bleeding, and what to do if bleeding occurs.

---

* Initially developed by Gordon J. Vanscoy, PharmD, MBA, University of Pittsburgh Medical Center, Drug Information and Pharmacoepidemiology Center. Revised for geriatric population by Laurie Jacobs, MD, and the American Geriatrics Society (AGS) Clinical Practice Committee. For further information call the AGS at (212) 308–1414.

6
PART

At the End of Life

Life is eternal; and love is immortal; and death is only a horizon; and a horizon is nothing save the limit of our sight.
Rossiter Worthington Raymond, 1840–1918

*For certain is death for the born
And certain is birth for the dead;
Therefore over the inevitable
Thou shouldst not grieve.*
Bhagavad-Gita, 250 BCE–AD 250 (approx.)

A man's dying is more the survivors' affair than his own.
Thomas Mann, 1875–1955

For love is strong as death.
Song of Solomon 8:6

For dying, you always have time.
Jewish Proverb

20
CHAPTER

Caring for the Terminally Ill Patient

THE DEVELOPMENT OF HOSPICE CARE

1879	The Sisters of Charity open hospices in Dublin.
1905	The Sisters of Charity open hospices in London.
1958–1965	Dr. Cicely Saunders works in St. Joseph's Hospice in London.
1967	Dr. Cicely Saunders opens St. Christopher's Hospice in South London.
1974	First American hospice opened in Connecticut.
1979	The National Hospice Organization formed in the United States.
1983	Congress passes Medicare Hospice Benefit.
1988	The Academy of Hospice Physicians formed in the United States.

Recent studies show that the nation's approximately 3000 hospice programs care for 15% of dying Americans—about 390,000 per year. Experts in end-of-life care consider that 30% to 40% of dying Americans could benefit from hospice-type terminal care, and it has even been suggested that the general hospice principles that will be discussed in this chapter would help anyone dying of a chronic illness, which means about 70% of the dying.

THE HOSPICE MINDSET

Webster's dictionary has two definitions of hospice:

1. Hospice, a program, begun in England in 1967, that eases the last days of terminally ill patients and assures a natural death in as home-like surroundings as possible. There are currently almost 1,500 hospice programs in the U.S.
2. Hospice, a building, usually kept by a religious order, where travelers can obtain rest and food.

PEARL: Those of us who now practice hospice care regard it as a state of mind more than a program or place. I call this the hospice mindset. Care of the terminally ill ideally should involve a team of experienced health professionals who work with the patient, family, and friends. The team members vary according to the availability of funds and interest among health professionals, but the key person is the hospice nurse, closely followed by the medical social worker. Consultation, as needed, with a dietician, a pharmacist, and physical and occupational therapists is helpful. Volunteers also can contribute a great deal in day-to-day patient care and family support. On occasion, with the patient's permission, they can even attend team meetings. A physician, serving as medical director, consults with and advises the team members and makes home visits as needed. If the patient is religious, a minister, priest, or rabbi, though not usually a member of the team, can provide counsel and spiritual comfort to the patient and often can give valuable insights to the hospice team.

The patient's home, a good nursing home, or a special hospice unit is the best setting for an easy, peaceful death. The worst place for a dying patient is the noisy, high-tech, emergency-oriented acute hospital. But even there, the problems of the dying patient can be effectively solved by a dedicated health professional who is familiar with the guidelines in this section of the book. Symptom management is the same no matter what the setting, and other, less knowledgeable acute-care staff can benefit from observing the hospice mindset in action.

By the time terminal care is needed, the diagnosis is not in doubt. Cure is not possible. The patient is sick, weak, and lacking in energy. He or she is likely to be suffering and may be in pain. (Pain and suffering are not the same, as will be explained.) Remember that death can come at any age—not only the old die.

The first step toward developing the hospice mindset is the realization *and acceptance* that none of us escape death. It is the inevitable end of life for every human, not just the terminally ill patient; in a sense we are all "terminal." Willingness to acknowledge this and to explore our own attitudes and concerns about dying and death allows progression to the next step in effective terminal care: the implementation of the following positive, dynamic management goals:

- To offer care, support, and love to the patient and family before, during, and after death
- To evaluate the whole person and relieve symptoms (pain, nausea, constipation, and so on) as they occur
- To address depression and suffering, both mental and spiritual, with love, patience, counseling, and judicious use of medications
- To give appropriate nutrition and hydration as wished by the patient

Some terminally ill patients and families come to me fearful and questioning because they are under the impression that hospice is totally negative, that all medications and other therapies are stopped immediately and the patient is just allowed to die. I take time to make it clear to them that this is far from the truth—any medication that is making the patient feel better will be continued. I describe to them the positive, immensely therapeutic aspects of good terminal care and how committed my team and I are to the concept of quality time for the patient, however long or short it might be, in whatever setting the patient finds himself or herself.

The terminally ill person must remain in control to the greatest degree possible, must be listened to, and must be treated with respect. If he or she becomes too sick to communicate easily, previously expressed wishes must be followed. Hospice patients must have a written "Do Not Attempt to Resuscitate" order in the event of death, for obvious reasons.

Hospice is not just for the elderly or cancer patients. Any terminally ill person, at any age, in any setting, can benefit from this kind of care. Since the onset of the AIDS epidemic, more young people and their caregivers are seeking hospice care. Unfortunately, many Americans who could benefit from this care never receive it for several reasons: many doctors see referral to hospice as an admission of defeat, and are reluctant to recommend stopping treatment even when it is clear that it is no longer effective. Patients and family members can share this attitude and have difficulty accepting that death is moving closer. The 40 million uninsured Americans have no chance of receiving hospice care. Health insurance companies vary in the amount of terminal care they will cover. Medicare reimbursement rules and punitive audits looking for fraud pose a considerable threat to hospice programs because a doctor is supposed to refer to them only patients with less than 6 months to live. This can be a difficult judgment call. Some diseases, such as end stage chronic obstructive lung disease and Parkinson's disease, deteriorate at unpredictable rates. And, as mentioned previously, the perception that hospice care is negative is still pervasive throughout the medical and lay community.

INTERACTIONS WITH THE PATIENT

The following rules can be applied in any setting—home, skilled nursing facility (SNF), or acute hospital. Your patients will remember your courtesy and kindness if you follow these rules.

- **PEARL: *Do not* give bad news over the telephone.** Arrange to meet your patient in a private place.
- Acknowledge to your patient that the situation is tragic and disturbing and you do not know why this has happened to him or her.

- Show respect for your patient by listening to him or her, making eye contact (if culturally acceptable), and treating the patient with courtesy.
- Touch your patient. The "laying on of hands" by the physician is one of medicine's oldest remedies, and comforts patients who may feel that they are too disgusting to be looked at or touched.
- Learn the value of listening in silence. Practice this. Let the patient and family members ventilate as needed.
- If the patient has a religious belief, even if you don't share it, support it and use it to help. **PEARL: If the patient has no religious belief, do not impose your beliefs on the patient. Neither preach nor proselytize; neither try to convert nor convince. *Listen and comfort only.***
- If the patient's faith takes a guilty or punitive form (for example, if he or she thinks disease and death are deserved as punishment for real or imagined sins), try to find a minister, priest, or rabbi experienced in hospice care to help, counsel, and comfort.
- Learn about and respect your patient's social and cultural background. Try to understand his or her viewpoint and use it to help where possible. The hospice team should identify key people in the family and culture and make allies of them.
- **PEARL: Apply the golden rule—*identify.*** Ask yourself "If I were dying, what would I want from my doctor, nurses, caregivers?"
- With the patient's permission, involve others who might help—family, friends, clergy, hospice organization, medical social worker, and financial or legal advisor.
- Learn about the grieving process. The patient is grieving before death; the survivors are grieving both before and after death. Know the stages of grieving:

  1. Denial
  2. Anger
  3. Bargaining
  4. Depression
  5. Acceptance

Some patients reach a final stage beyond these five, which I call the "good-bye" stage, in which they are able to call in loved ones, talk with them, and say good-bye. This can start the healing of the wounds that we all give each other throughout life, and can make grieving easier after death.

INTERACTIONS WITH CAREGIVERS

- **Do not** give information about your patient to other family members or friends without his or her permission. Even within a seemingly close family, confidentiality must be respected. An exception to this rule would be if the patient were comatose or mentally unable to understand the diagnosis and its implications for treatment and end-of-life decisions. Even here, care is needed: following the strictest letter of the law, such information should be given only to the person designated in the patient's Durable Power of Attorney for Health Care (see Chap. 23). Most people do not have such a document, however, so in this situation I use my judgment and communicate with the spouse or the family member who seems closest to the patient. It is helpful to identify one such key person in the family with whom you communicate most often. This person then relays information to the other members as needed.
- The physician should participate in family conferences, whether in the home, SNF, or acute hospital. Although the other members of the hospice team are valued and respected by the family, considerable weight is put on the doctor's comments. What the physician says will be long remembered, favorably or unfavorably.
- Show that you care. Accept that in some cases fear and anger about the illness will be directed at you. Learn to let this wash over you without harming you. Express your feelings to the other hospice team members and benefit from their support.
- Be prepared to answer questions such as "How will death come?" "What will it be like? A struggle,

peaceful, a coma?" (See "Answering Questions" in this chapter, and Chap. 21.)

FAMILY DYNAMICS

Family dysfunction is common around the death of a family member, whether he or she was loved, feared, hated, or any combination of these. The hospice team can help to improve family dynamics and deflect some of the anger or guilt away from the attending physician; the doctor can be more helpful to the patient by remaining uninvolved in such family emotional storms. (This is one of the most difficult tests for the health professional—to be involved and caring with the patient, yet take no emotional part in difficult family and interpersonal interactions.)

A common event is the arrival of a close relative who has lost touch with the dying person. Full of remorse and anger, this person may demand that "Everything must be done!" It takes time and patience to deal with this person and explain that the hospice plans are the patient's wish and are justified by the situation.

The death of an elderly person, though sad, lacks the sense of injustice felt when a young person dies. People will say of the elder, "At least he or she had a good life." Viewing the dead body, mourning rituals, the funeral, and the coming together of family and friends can all help toward acceptance of this sad event. The concept of a celebration of the person's life, instead of a funeral, is gaining ground. I have attended a few of these and found them positive and inspiring, and the family and friends in each case were uplifted.

Nevertheless, sadness after any loss is a normal reaction and can be intense at anniversaries and formerly shared holidays such as Thanksgiving and Christmas. Support groups in many communities can help the survivors.

Allowing the survivor to talk about the loss can help toward some resolution of conflicts and regrets. The loving presence of family and friends can be a great consolation. If grieving continues indefinitely at a level of intensity that impairs function, psychiatric help may be essential to avoid the real risk of major depression, which can end in suicide. (See Chap. 12.)

OTHER ISSUES

Laboratory Testing

I do not do any "routine" tests on my hospice patients. (See Chap. 5.) The terminally ill always have abnormal labs. Attempts to normalize them will fail and may harm the patient. I order tests only if I am convinced that the results will improve therapy and the patient's comfort. For example, hypercalcemia can cause nausea, so a patient could benefit from having it treated. Much clinical judgment is needed here. Talk with more experienced hospice health professionals if in doubt.

Your Attitudes

Examine your own attitudes toward death and dying—your own death, the death of parents, children, friends, patients, pets. Are you suppressing feelings of anger, anxiety, or guilt associated with death? Do you always see death as a professional and even a personal defeat? Have you seen anyone die a natural, peaceful death away from the hospital?

It can help to talk through some of these issues with an experienced hospice worker (either medical, religious, or volunteer) when you are starting out in this field. You will be reassured to find that you are not alone if you have problems with death and dying.

Pain Versus Suffering

Be aware that pain and suffering are not the same. Suffering is more than pain, though pain may be a part of it. Feelings of powerlessness, loss, isolation, rotting away, and looking and feeling unattractive can overwhelm the patient dying of an incurable disease. He or she may worry about family and finances or unfinished business, and may feel guilt, anger, or fear of the unknown. All these and more are components of suffering and all are made worse by uncontrolled pain.

Pain can be controlled. Suffering can be lessened by the hospice team working together with the patient, caregivers, friends, volunteers, and religious support. The practitioner who tries to do all this alone will fail and end up burned out. The members of the hospice team support each other as well as the patient.

Answering Questions

The patient and caregivers usually ask, "How long, Doctor?" This is one of the hardest questions to answer. Studies have shown that even hospice experts have difficulty estimating how long a patient has left to live. All you can say is that in your experience, cases similar to this have lived for x number of days, weeks, or months, but you should point out that every human being is different. If they have their own reasons, even the desperately ill can survive for a surprising length of time. The converse of this is the patient who decides he or she has had enough, turns his or her face to the wall, and dies sooner than expected.

Caregivers, and occasionally the patient, might ask "What will it be like, Doctor?" When you hear this question, it is a good idea to ask the inquirers what they expect. Often you will find that they are worried because they have heard horror stories about agonizing deaths. You will be able to reassure them that the good hospice care you and your team will provide will not let this happen. It is important to take time and listen to fears and worries.

FINAL WORDS

Take to heart the advice in this chapter and apply this hospice mindset as needed to all your terminal patients. They will be better off for it, and you will become a skilled practitioner of the healing, caring art of medicine.

21
CHAPTER

Signs of Approaching Death

*Death be not proud, though some have
called thee
Mighty and dreadful. . . .
One short sleep past, we wake eternally,
And death shall be no more; death, thou shalt die.*
John Donne, 1572–1631

The changes listed in this chapter reveal the body preparing for the final stages of life, which lead to death. They can occur hours or days before death, and they do not appear at the same time or in any regular order. Some may never appear at all—each person is unique in both living and dying.

- Limbs become cool to the touch. Lividity develops. Blood circulation slows.
- Body temperature can fluctuate. Cool sponging, aspirin (ASA), or acetaminophen can help fever and sweating.
- Sleep time increases and the patient may become difficult to arouse. This is normal in the dying patient. It is good for the family and friends to take

turns sitting with the patient. Silence is fine. Just being there, perhaps holding his or her hand, is enough.

- Periods of confusion may occur or increase, and even close family may not be recognized.
- The patient may become restless and disoriented, and can have visual and auditory hallucinations.
- Incontinence of bowel and bladder may occur. Urinary output decreases and eventually stops.
- The patient usually has neither appetite nor thirst. He or she has lost interest in eating and drinking. This is normal and is not painful. Attempts to force nutrition or hydration on the dying patient have been shown to *cause* discomfort—for example, gastric distention, nausea, and diarrhea. Tube feedings are contraindicated. **PEARL: Even if the dying patient is not eating, you should continue good mouth care, which makes the patient more comfortable.** If medications are still needed, crush them or give them parenterally, but re-evaluate whether they are really needed. Are you treating the patient or yourself?
- Pooling of saliva and excessive secretions may cause noisy, gurgling breathing. The patient is too weak by now to cough up secretions, causing distress to the observers but not to the patient. If family members are very upset by these sounds, you can dry up secretions. (See Other Troublesome Symptoms, Chap. 22.)
- Acuity of hearing and clarity of vision may decrease. Speech may become difficult. **PEARL: Hearing is the last of the senses to be lost, so make sure that all conversations are appropriate for the patient to hear.**
- Breathing may become irregular, with periods of apnea and Cheyne-Stokes breathing. When this happens, the patient is no longer aware of it. Reassure the family that the patient is not suffering or disturbed by the irregular breathing.
- Some patients slip into a coma followed by death. Others remain conscious until close to the end.

22
CHAPTER

Symptom Management in the Terminally Ill Patient

Good symptom control is the patient's right and the physician's duty.
Anonymous

In the last stages of a final illness, we need only the absence of pain and the presence of family.
Helen Hayes, with Marion Glasserow Gladney,
Loving Life (1987)

PAIN

Pain is the most common and feared symptom, suffered by 65% to 85% of hospice cancer patients and present in two or more sites in 80% of terminally ill patients. The pain is usually caused by underlying organic lesions and the patient can have more than one kind of pain. Identifying the *sources* of pain is crucial to its effective management.

Approach to the Patient with Pain

Identify Sources of Pain

- **Visceral involvement** with tumor infiltration and some degree of inflammation. Can be referred to body surface. Responds well to narcotics.
- **Bone metastases** respond less well to narcotics alone. Add nonsteroidal anti-inflammatory drugs (NSAIDs) to the narcotic. If still not controlled, add corticosteroids (discussed later). In some cases, palliative irradiation can help.
- **Neuritic involvement** (dysthesias, lancinating pain) responds well to narcotics combined with tricyclics. The next choices are carbamazepine, phenytoin, or mexiletine.
- **Mucosal pain**. Look for a cause such as candidiasis and treat it. Avoid mouthwashes with alcohol. Good oral hygiene is essential for the patient's comfort.
- **Hollow viscus pain** (cramping, colicky in nature). Try an anticholinergic such as hyoscyamine, oxybutynin, or suppositories of belladonna and opioid. These can be used in combination with other pain medications. Check for fecal impaction and urinary retention.

Achieve Pain Control

Pain, the memory of pain, and the anticipation of pain bring anxiety, depression, fear, and misery. Medication must be given *round the clock* at regular intervals to keep pain under control, with additional doses for breakthrough pain. Anticipate pain and keep it under control. Reassess often.

PEARL: There is no place in hospice-type care for as-needed (prn) medication alone.

Start by evaluating *all* medications being taken, including prescription, nonprescription, and alternative medicinal preparations. Anticipate side effects. You might have to treat the side effects rather than discontinue the medication causing them.

Listen to your patient: the pain is what, where, and how severe he or she says it is. Ask the patient to rate the intensity of pain on a scale of 0 to 5, with 5 the most severe. This number can be entered on a chart to track the effectiveness of treatment.

Review all previous analgesics used. How much of each was the patient taking? How effective were they?

PEARL: In this setting, there is no optimal narcotic dose, nor is there a maximum narcotic dose. Some patients get relief from as little as 5 mg oral morphine every 4 hours, whereas others need as much as 1500 mg every 4 hours to control the pain. Be prepared to reassure your patient and caregivers that addiction does not occur in the terminally ill patient. The medications are being used to control pain, not to "get high."

Be prepared to discuss drug tolerance with your patient. Many patients fear that, "If I use the medicine now, it won't work when I really need it." Reassure them that this is unlikely, and that if it does happen, it can be managed successfully.

A schedule of long-acting narcotics may achieve effective pain control as well as short-acting drugs. For example, you might prescribe sustained-release morphine sulphate (MS) Contin every 12 hours, plus oral MS every 4 to 6 hours for breakthrough pain. Titrate the dosages until pain control is satisfactory. Sometimes adequate doses of the narcotic must be accompanied by non-narcotic medications to achieve effective control.

Use nonmedication treatments such as a hospital bed, special mattress, or Foley catheter to improve the patient's comfort. Music, massage, relaxation techniques, hypnosis, meditation, and prayer can all help. Keep an open mind about possible benefits of alternative medicines and therapies and respect their importance to the patient and family.

If pain is proving difficult to manage, do not be reluctant to consult with colleagues who have expertise in caring for the dying. Anesthesiologists are another source of helpful ideas. For instance, intraspinal infusion and nerve blocks are often effective.

Be aware of the downward spiral that can occur. Anxiety, guilt, and a sense of helplessness and fear make pain worse, and pain causes anxiety and fear.

The sleepless patient may brood and worry in the solitary hours of darkness. Sedation can be appropriate. Lorazepam (Ativan) can help in this situation. In some patients, a small dose (25 mg) of trazodone (Desyrel) at bedtime helps.

Analgesics in Common Use

The commonly used analgesics can be divided into non-narcotics, weak narcotics, and narcotics. **PEARL: It is better to know a small number of analgesics thoroughly than a larger number less well.**

Non-Narcotics

Non-narcotic analgesics include acetaminophen, aspirin preparations (ASA), and NSAIDs. You can start with these and then move to narcotics, or you can combine them with narcotics if pain is not controlled. Adjust ASA dosage in cachectic patients with low albumin. ASA and acetaminophen are equivalent in antipyretic and analgesic effects. Acetaminophen lacks anti-inflammatory and anti-prostaglandin effects. If these are needed, ASA or NSAIDs should be used, with vigilance for side effects, especially in very old patients. (See Chap. 17.)

Weak Narcotics

Codeine preparations, oxycodone, and hydrocodone have limited use because of a clinical "ceiling effect"—after 2 or 3 upward dose adjustments, side effects increase more than the analgesic effect. If one of these is failing to control pain, do not add another weak narcotic to it. Discontinue the ineffective drug and move up to a narcotic.

Narcotics

Adequate doses of oral narcotics can control 80% to 90% of pain. When using liquid oral narcotics, measure with a syringe, not a kitchen spoon. Never start a narcotic without laxative cover. Senokot-S (1–4 tablets by mouth daily) is the current favorite, or you can ask patients if they have a favorite laxative.

When a patient's pain has been inadequately controlled, and he or she has been anxious, fearful, sleepless, and exhausted for some time, relieving the pain can cause him or her to sleep for long periods. This is not a cause for worry.

Morphine Sulfate

The most useful, most commonly used narcotic is morphine sulfate (MS). It is effective orally as liquid or tablets, and is absorbed from the oral mucosa as well as the gastrointestinal tract. It can be given subcutaneously (SC), intramuscularly (IM), intravenously (IV), epidurally, and by rectal suppository. The oral dose of MS is three to six times the parenteral dose. Start with 10 to 20 mg of oral MS every 4 hours and titrate upward to pain control (Table 22–1). Whatever dose was needed for breakthrough pain should be added to the next regular dose until the pain is under control. Remember, there is no optimal dose and no maximum dose. When the pain is controlled, the patient can be switched to MS Contin every 12 hours, using the same dose in 24 hours as the shorter-acting MS total, supplemented as needed with shorter-acting MS for breakthrough pain. Hospice workers find that once the pain is under control, the regular dose often can be reduced and the patient will remain pain free. Know this medication well.

Subcutaneous or Intravenous Pump

If the oral approach does not work, MS can be given SC via a programmable pump that can inject up to 1 mL per hour. (The MS solution can be made up in different strengths, with a maximum concentration of 50 mg per mL.) Calculate the total oral dose of morphine in 24 hours and divide by 3 to 6 for parenteral administration. The pump can be programmed to administer a continuous dose with additional patient-controlled boluses. Other kinds of drugs, such as haloperidol (a major tranquilizer) and metoclopramide (useful in treating gastroesophageal reflux, gastroparesis, and nausea), can also be administered using the same pump, avoiding an additional injection. A typical pump order would read:

MS 5 mg per hour continuously SC, with 2-mg bolus up to twice hourly.

If SC administration does not work, move to IV. Use a plan similar to that for the SC pump, with programmable IV delivery of comparable doses of MS.

Other Narcotics

In the MS-intolerant patient, **hydromorphone (Dilaudid)** is the best option. It is approximately four times as potent orally as MS, with a similar duration of action. It can be given IM, IV, SC, and by rectal suppository.

Fentanyl (Duragesic) patches (Table 22–2) are available in 25, 50, 75, and 100 µg/hr delivery systems. The patches last 3 days, with steady-state levels being reached 5 to 6 days after first application and after each dosage change. Speedy dose adjustments—titration upwards to control pain—are not possible, and the upper limit of dose in terminally ill patients is 200 µg per hour. Above this, side effects outweigh benefits. Side effects include nausea and vomiting, itching, hypoventilation, confusion, constipation, and urinary retention. Most hospice physicians prescribe fentanyl patches only occasionally. Absorption is unpredictable in dying patients, so it is difficult to give doses equivalent to oral MS. Exposure to an external heat source can speed up the release of opioid from the patch.

When I have terminally ill patients using fentanyl patches whose pain is poorly controlled, I start them off on oral MS and titrate this up while reducing the patch strength every 3 days and then discontinuing it. I then use MS as described.

Although not generally helpful in dying patients with moderate to severe pain, these patches can be useful in more functional patients with mild to moderate chronic pain.

Table 22–1. DOSAGES OF ORAL ANALGESICS THAT ACHIEVE PAIN RELIEF COMPARABLE TO 10–20 MG ORAL MORPHINE SULFATE

Medication	Dose (mg)	Dosage Interval (hr)	Oral:Parenteral Ratio	Comments
Morphine (Roxanol) MS Contin, Oramorph SR	**10–20** 30–60	**Q 4** Q 12	**3–6:1**	**First choice** Slow onset of action. Never use prn. For maintenance *only* when acute pain has been controlled with short-acting MS. Can use rectally.
Hydromorphone (Dilaudid)	2–4	Q 4	5:1	IM, IV, SC, rectal suppositories available: same dose as oral. Euphorigenic. More soluble than MS. Available in high-potency injectable form 10 mg/mL.
Levorphano (Levo-Dromoran)	2	Q 4–6	2:1	Long half-life (12–16 hr). Accumulation can make titration difficult.
Methadone (Dolophine)	2.5–5	Q 6–8	2:1	Long half-life. Accumulation makes titration difficult. More respiratory depression than MS. Receptor blockade prevents use of supplemental MS.

Drug	Dose	Frequency	Ratio	Comments
Meperidine (Demerol)	50	Q 2–3	4:1	Don't use this—too difficult to titrate. Poor oral absorption, short half-life. High incidence of toxic effects, including convulsions, at higher dosage levels.
Hydrocodone (Vicodin has acetaminophen added)	5–10	Q 4	2:1	Can work for moderate pain. Effective cough suppressant.
Oxycodone (Percocet has acetaminophen added; Percodan has ASA added.)	5–10	Q 4	2:1	Short-acting. Moderate pain. Works better combined with ASA or acetaminophen.
Pentazocine (Talwin)	50	Q 3–4	3:1	Best avoided. Psychotic effects with higher doses. Relatively short duration of action. Nausea, vomiting, blurred vision, drowsiness, hallucinations.
Propoxyphene (Darvocet-N 100 has acetaminophen added; Darvon; Darvon Compound-65)	65–100	Q 4		Best avoided. Long half-life, low potency, and small dosage range. Nausea, vomiting, dizziness, drowsiness common.

IM = intramuscular; IV = intravenous; MS = morphine sulfate; SC = subcutaneous.

**Table 22–2. FENTANYL 72-HOUR
TRANSDERMAL SYSTEM: APPROXIMATE
COMPARABLE MS DOSE**

Fentanyl	Comparable Total MS Dose in 24 Hours
25-µg patch	45–134 mg
50-µg patch	135–224 mg
75-µg patch	225–314 mg
100-µg patch	315–404 mg
200-µg patch	675–764 mg

See also comments in text.

Useful Adjuncts to Analgesics

As already mentioned, other types of medication and other therapies often are helpful adjuncts to analgesics in effectively controlling pain. The following entries are listed in the order of frequency with which I prescribe them.

Antidepressants

Tricyclics are useful in neurogenic pain. They have long half-lives. A sedating tricyclic such as amitriptyline (25–75 mg), given at bedtime, can give a good night's sleep, improve mood, and enhance analgesia. (See Table 12–1 for further information. The information in this table applies to frail, sick, adult patients of all ages.)

Other antidepressants also are proving useful in pain control for some patients. (See Chap. 12.)

Anticonvulsants

Anticonvulsants are the second choice (after tricyclics) to control neurogenic pain. Usually a loading dose is not needed.

Dextroamphetamine (Dexedrine)

Amphetamine derivatives potentiate analgesics, so that the narcotic dose can be lowered and somnolence reduced. They are also antidepressant. They are given orally at a dose of 5 mg in the morning and at lunchtime.

Methylphenidate (Ritalin)

Ritalin is a useful alternative to dextroamphetamine, with similar effects. It is given orally at a dose of 5 to 10 mg in the morning and at lunchtime.

Corticosteroids

Corticosteroids can be useful for patients with brain, bone, and liver metastases; nerve or spinal cord compression; or hypercalcemia. They reduce elevated intracranial pressure and help associated nausea and vomiting. They can also temporarily improve appetite and mood, and reduce sweating and fever.

Start with prednisone 1–2 mg/kg, tapering over 2 to 3 weeks to a maintenance dose of 10 to 15 mg daily.

Dexamethasone (Decadron) can be used in a similar way: 0.75 mg of dexamethasone is equivalent to 5 mg of prednisone.

Haloperidol (Haldol)

Haloperidol has some analgesic effect, can be sedating, has anti-anxiety and antidepressant effects, and can help the dysphoria sometimes caused by narcotics. It is useful in terminal demented or delirious patients, especially at night. It can be combined with narcotics and antidepressants.

The oral dose is 0.5 to 5 mg twice daily (BID), three times daily (TID), or four times daily (QID). It can also be given IM or SC, or by a subcutaneous pump, at similar dosages.

Naloxone (Narcan)

Narcotic-induced respiratory depression can be reversed by 0.4 mg of naloxone in 10 mL, given IV, IM, or SC in small boluses.

Heroin

Heroin is not available for prescription in the United States, but is available in Britain, with special license, for pain control. The oral form seems to have no advantages over MS in most (but not all) patients. In a very small number of patients, the injectable form, which is more absorbable than other injected narcotics, gives more effective pain control than any other medication.

Other Therapies

Relaxation therapy, acupuncture, biofeedback, hypnosis, TENS, meditation, and massage all can contribute to pain management. Alcohol can add to the effects of some medications and oppose others. Even though it can be anti-analgesic, if a drink was part of the patient's previous routine and he or she enjoys it, I would support continuing the routine.

NAUSEA AND VOMITING

Many patients say that constant nausea is worse than pain. It is important to control this symptom, even by carefully combining two or more anti-emetic medications. Watch for side effects.

Identify the Cause

First try to determine the cause:

- Disorders of the gastrointestinal tract.

  - Gastric stasis secondary to disease or medications.
  - Pressure on the stomach from organomegaly or tumor ("squashed stomach").
  - Partial or complete obstruction. Treat this conservatively in a dying patient.
  - Constipation or fecal impaction. Yes, this can cause nausea and vomiting.

- Medications and other therapies.

  - Narcotics
  - Digoxin
  - ASA
  - Radiation and chemotherapy

- Electrolyte imbalance, especially hypercalcemia.
- Raised intracranial pressure. Radiation therapy might help, or corticosteroids in doses as already described.

Medications to Control Nausea and Vomiting

PEARL: Antiemetics may have to be given on a regular dosing schedule rather than prn, and a combination of two or more may be needed to control nausea. (Table 22–3). If your patient still has intractable nausea or vomiting after a reasonable trial of these medications, talk with an anesthesiologist, who will suggest a number of other effective injectable preparations. The medications are listed here in the order of frequency with which I prescribe them.

Prochlorperazine (Compazine)

IM, IV, or rectal suppositories work better than oral medications when the nausea has no obvious mechanical reason such as ileus. It doesn't make sense to put medications in the stomach of a patient with nausea and vomiting, but if the vomiting, or the trigger for it, can be anticipated, an oral dose, IM injection, or a suppository given 30 to 60 minutes beforehand can work.

Trimethobenzamide (Tigan)

This drug is available for oral or IM administration, or as rectal suppositories. Its indications and use are similar to those of prochlorperazine.

TABLE 22–3. MEDICATIONS THAT CONTROL NAUSEA AND VOMITING

Medication	PO	PR	IM, SC, IV
Chlorpromazine (Thorazine)	10–25 mg Q 4–6 hr	50–100 mg suppository Q 6–8 hr prn	IM: 12.5–25 mg initially, then if no hypotension 12.5–50 mg TID–QID
Cisapride (Propulsid)	10 mg up to QID		
Dimenhydrinate (Dramamine)	50–100 mg Q 4–8 hr up to a maximum of 400 mg daily		IM, IV: 50 mg prn
Lorazepam (Ativan)	0.5–2 mg BID–TID up to maximum of 6 mg in 24 hr		IM: 0.5–4 mg
Metoclopramide (Reglan)	5–15 mg TID–QID		IM, SC: 5–10 mg IV: 0.5–2mg/kg given over 30 min
Prochlorperazine (Compazine)	5–10 mg TID–QID, prn or on a regular dosing schedule. Long-acting: 10–15 mg in am or 10 mg BID.	25mg BID	IM: 5–10 mg Q 4–6 hr up to maximum of 40 mg in 24 hr
Promethazine (Phenergan)	12.5–25 mg BID–QID	12.5–25 mg BID–QID	IM: 12.5–25 mg BID–QID
Trimethobenzamide (Tigan)	250 mg TID–QID	200 mg TID–QID	IM: 200 mg TID–QID

IM = intramuscular; IV = intravenous; PO = by mouth; PR = by rectum; SC = subcutaneous.
See also comments in text.

Transderm Scopolamine Patch

Developed for travel sickness, this patch works well in centrally induced nausea and vomiting. Watch out for dry mouth and constipation. This patch can cause confusion or disorientation in debilitated patients. A new patch is used every 3 days.

Lorazepam (Ativan)

The oral or sublingual forms of lorazepam are useful to help anxiety, agitation, and insomnia as well as nausea. The injectable form can produce amnesia, so I seldom prescribe it.

Corticosteroids

Used either alone or in combination with other antinausea medications, corticosteroids can provide some degree of relief. Use the same dosage schedule as when used as an adjunct to analgesics, or prescribe a maintenance dose.

Metoclopramide (Reglan)

Metoclopramide is useful for nausea caused by a tumor or drug-related ileus. *Check for fecal impaction.* If the patient is on a pump, this drug can be added to the mixture and given SC or IV.

Tetrahydrocannabinol

Tetrahydrocannabinol is one of the active principles in marijuana. I have prescribed the oral form—Marinol—and most of my patients found it ineffective. The inhaled smoke is effective in 70% of users. It can produce euphoria. (Surely in the dying patient this is good.) Side effects are mild—dizziness, somnolence, dysphoria. It is now legal to suggest this form of therapy to your patient in California, but is still against federal law, and the DEA has threatened to pursue and even prosecute physicians who try to help their patients control their symptoms in this way.

Cisapride (Propulsid)

This drug helps nausea and vomiting in some patients.

Chlorpromazine (Thorazine)

Use chlorpromazine with great care in elderly patients. It is sedating and tranquilizing, and can drop blood pressure. It helps in some cases of intractable hiccups. It is available in oral, injectable, and rectal forms.

Dimenhydrinate (Dramamine)

Used to treat motion sickness, this drug helps nausea in some patients. The oral preparation is sold without a prescription. Watch for anticholinergic side effects.

Promethazine (Phenergan)

This drug works against nausea in some patients. In some it can be anti-analgesic, and its sedative effect can add to other sedating drugs being prescribed. Watch for anticholinergic side effects. It can be given orally, IM, or rectally. IM injection must be deep. SC injection can result in tissue necrosis.

ANXIETY AND DEPRESSION

PEARL: Counseling, reassurance, and practical help in putting affairs in order are important ways to combat anxiety and depression. If medication is also needed, some of the drugs used to help in the control of pain or nausea may be used. See the preceding discussions for more specific information.

- **Antidepressants**. Bicyclics, tricyclics, tetracyclics, or newer agents may be used. Agitated depression is not uncommon and can be difficult to diagnose. (See Chap. 12 and Table 12–1.)
- **Lorazepam** (Ativan)

- **Dextroamphetamine** (Dexedrine). This drug (oral only) potentiates the effects of narcotics and opposes drowsiness, as well as being an anti-depressant.
- **Propanolol** (Inderal). This is nonsedating and works well in suppressing anxiety in some patients. It is good for panic disorder. The dosage is up to 40 mg four times daily (QID). A longer-acting preparation can be given in a single dose: atenolol 50–200 mg daily (QD), at bedtime (HS).
- **Haloperidol** (Haldol). Can be very useful.
- **Thioridizine** (Mellaril) can be helpful in severe anxiety and agitation. It is more sedating than haloperidol. It can be given only orally, at a dose of 10 to 50 mg BID to QID. Sometimes, but rarely, a higher dose can be used, but watch for sedation, somnolence, and anticholinergic effects.
- **Chlorpromazine** (Thorazine)
- **Midazolam** (Versed) can be given orally, IM, IV, and SC. It can be combined with haloperidol. It is sedating and should be used with great care because of respiratory depression or arrest. I would not use this without the help of an anesthesiologist.
- **Barbiturates** are generally not useful in terminally ill patients because they can be anti-analgesic and can produce paradoxical excitement. The exception to this rule is the use of a 200-mg Nembutal suppository to relieve excessive restlessness in the dying patient.

OTHER TROUBLESOME SYMPTOMS

- **Dehydration** occurs in the dying patient. It is not painful or unpleasant. IVs are not indicated because they can cause dyspnea, immobilize a limb, and decrease the comfort of the terminally ill patient. Good mouth care is essential to keep the oral mucosa moist and clean and to comfort the patient.
- **Diarrhea** can be treated by giving loperamide (Imodium) in the usual way after each loose stool, up to 6 in 24 hours, or 2 or 3 times daily. If that is

ineffective, give Lomotil 1 by mouth after each loose stool up to 6 in 24 hours, or on a regular schedule 2 or 3 times daily.

- **Dyspnea** is frightening for the patient and can produce panic attacks. How would it feel to be drowning in air? Give oxygen prn (2–4 liters/min, or more if needed) via nasal cannula or mask. Small doses of MS given around the clock are helpful. Bronchodilators, antibiotics, diuretics, and minor tranquilizers can all be tried.

- **Fever.** Use 650 mg of acetaminophen (Tylenol) orally (liquid or tablets) or rectally every 6 hours for temperature > 101°F (38.3°C).

- **Hiccups**. Intractable hiccups can be difficult to influence. Try chlorpromazine 10–50 mg orally (po) TID or QID. If there is no improvement after a day or so, try giving 10–50 mg IM. Phenytoin (Dilantin, 100mg every 8 hr) can be helpful in some cases. You also can try Reglan 10 mg QID.

- **Mouth problems**

  - For **dry mouth**, use a saline mouthwash of 1 teaspoon salt in 1 cup warm water. Also helpful are artificial saliva, glycerin-based mouthwashes, and ice chips (which can be flavored). Frequent, meticulous mouth care is important. Avoid alcohol-based mouth preparations.

  - Candidiasis is common in debilitated patients and is very painful. Treat it with any of the following:

    - Nystatin pastilles
    - Stanford-Kaiser mouthwash (tetracycline, nystatin, hydrocortisone, and water). Most hospital pharmacists know this, or a variation of it, and will make it up for your patients.
    - Ketoconazole (1 tablet daily)
    - Mycelex troches

  - For aphthous ulcers, amlexanox (Aphthasol) oral paste 5% dabbed onto the ulcer after meals and at bedtime helps in some patients. An old remedy is gentian violet aqueous solution applied to the ulcer TID. This is antiseptic and soothing, and I have seen it work in many patients.

- For herpetic ulcers, acyclovir systemically might help. A local treatment is amlexanox oral paste 5% after meals and at bedtime.

- For **wet or gurgling respirations**, use atropine solution (4 mg/mL, 0.2 mg/drop). Start with 0.2 mg sublingually (SL) or SC every 4 to 6 hours prn. This may be increased in 0.2-mg increments to a maximum dose of 1 mg SL or SC every 4 to 6 hours prn.

- **Loss of appetite** is often a concern of patients and their families. Megace is a synthetic progesterone derivative said to stimulate appetite. It usually has no lasting effect in the terminally ill patient. Similarly, corticosteroids can produce a brief, temporary improvement in appetite, but the effect does not last.

- **Weight loss** occurs before death. Its cause seems to be more than just loss of appetite. Perhaps decreased absorption and ineffective use of food, as well as the shutdown of liver and kidney function, play a large role. There is no effective treatment for this weight loss. **PEARL: Nasogastric or gastrostomy tube placement is not appropriate for the dying patient.** It can lead to aspiration pneumonia, self-extubation, use of restraints, bloating, nausea, and diarrhea.

- **Weakness and lack of energy**. Unfortunately, there is no effective treatment for the weakness and lack of energy that terminally ill people experience. All my hospice patients have asked me if there is any kind of "tonic" I could give them to boost their strength. There is none.

23

CHAPTER 23

Intensity of Treatment

Federal legislation called the Patient Self-Determination Act became law in the United States in December 1991. According to this law, institutions such as hospitals, nursing homes, home health agencies, hospices, and health maintenance organizations who are reimbursed by Medicare, Medicaid, or both, are required to inform patients about their rights to make health care decisions and about advance directives for care should the patients become too sick or injured to speak for themselves. As technology advances, it becomes more important for individuals to decide for themselves the degree of medical intervention that they want applied in case of illness or injury.

PEARL: Heroic procedures and treatments can be justified if the patient is likely to benefit from them and have a favorable outcome. Tests and procedures done from intellectual curiosity alone, or simply because they exist, cannot be justified. Quantity and quality of life are not the same, but they are not mutually exclusive.

With the technology now available, for example, we can resuscitate some patients who have died and keep them alive indefinitely with severe, irreversible brain damage. These patients live in a persistent vegetative state (PVS)—"The lights are on, but nobody's home." PVS is a tragedy for the survivors. The person will never recover, so there is no resolution and the family cannot mourn and then move on and continue with their lives. Because these patients remain comatose, they need total nursing care with gastrostomy or naso-gastric tube feedings and they have no control over bowel or bladder. Therefore it is almost impossible to have them at home. Many end up in nursing homes at great expense, which can wipe out the family's fi-nances. The very few who remain at home are main-tained there at considerable cost to the family and so-ciety.

If this person has not left an indication of his or her wishes for intensity of treatment in such circum-stances, family members can be reluctant to discon-tinue life support. This sad, futile picture reinforces the value of advance planning, in which serious deci-sions are made with due consideration and not at a time of crisis.

HEALTH CARE DECISIONS

PEARL: Each individual has the right at any time to ac-cept or refuse any form of medical treatment or testing. Therapy can be refused even if it might prolong life. Ben-efits and risks associated with every form of treatment should be presented to the patient, and where more than one kind of therapy is available, the relative mer-its of each should be discussed.

Using either a formal legal document or informal means, individuals can give instructions to be carried out if he or she becomes seriously ill and unable to make his or her wishes known. These instructions may be that life-prolonging measures should not be used if there is no likelihood of recovery, or that a particular treatment or type of life support (e.g., ventilator, naso-gastric tube) should be tried for a limited time and then discontinued if there is no good result. This latter plan sounds good in theory, but can be more difficult in practice, especially if family members misinterpret the ending of such futile treatments as killing the pa-tient. Ethics committees now exist in most hospitals to address such sad, difficult cases.

ADVANCE DIRECTIVES

Living Will

A living will is one of the ways that an individual can give instructions about his or her care. It is a written directive to family members and health professionals, generally stating that no extraordinary measures should be used to prolong life in the event of terminal illness or coma when there is no hope of improvement. All comfort and supportive care would be given. There are two kinds of living wills, statutory and non-statutory. In the statutory living will, a state law describes what the form must say and it does not allow the naming of a surrogate decision maker. A typical nonstatutory living will can be written in the person's own words and can have a space for naming a surrogate decision maker. However, the living will has not worked well in practice for the following reasons:

- The wording varies, particularly in the nonstatutory forms, and can be vague and ambiguous—What is meant by "terminally ill"? What is an "extraordinary measure"? These answers could vary according to circumstances.
- In many states a living will is not regarded as binding unless signed after a diagnosis of terminal or incurable illness has been made. This takes away the option of making a careful, well-considered decision about these matters before a crisis occurs.
- Some states require a specific form for a living will and do not accept one from another state.
- They are not accepted in every state.
- The non-statutory living will, although giving useful information about the patient's wishes, provides only minimal legal protection to the physician who acts on it.
- The statutory living will may give a physician more protection from liability, but it could be challenged legally by a dissatisfied family member. It is not unusual for a family member who has not been seen for years to turn up, full of remorse, when a patient is dying, and demand that

everything must be done! whether in the patient's best interests or not. Such people have brought lawsuits for wrongful death against health professionals. In such a case, the existence of a living will, either statutory or nonstatutory, would strengthen the case for the health professional who followed the patient's wishes. However, an experienced attorney can make even a competent, well-intentioned person look bad, and no one wants the messy, upsetting hassle of a lawsuit.

It is better to use a durable power of attorney for health care (DPAHC), which is clearer, more uniform, more widely accepted, and has more force in the law for both patient and physician.

Durable Power of Attorney for Health Care

A DPAHC is a document that gives authority to another adult to make decisions about medical treatments if the individual named in the DPAHC becomes incapacitated and unable to do so. A DPAHC is generally preferable to a living will; it is clearer, more uniform, and more widely accepted. Anyone of sound mind who is at least 18 years of age can fill out such a form. A lawyer is *not* needed to fill it out or make it legal. Many hospitals and medical societies can provide copies of a standard form.

The representative named on the DPAHC is not permitted to agree to certain treatments, including commitment to a mental hospital, electric shock treatment, or psychosurgery (a brain operation to change personality). The DPAHC also does not allow the surrogate to make financial decisions; it is for health care only.

The person making the DPAHC must talk with the chosen agent to be sure that the wishes expressed in it are clearly understood. The doctor should also be informed. A back-up person or persons should be named in case the chosen agent is not available.

Copies of this document should be given to the chosen representatives, other family members, any lawyer involved, and the attending physician. The original should be kept in a safe place with similar important documents.

The DPAHC form can also be used to record treatments that the individual wishes and does not wish to be carried out, without naming an agent. This does not have the same legal standing as the full DPAHC because no agent is named, but it is still a valuable indication of the person's wishes.

The DPAHC remains in effect indefinitely unless the form used has a stated time limit, in some cases 7 years. A different period of time can be specified. It can be changed or revoked at any time by the person making it, as long as the revised wishes can be communicated.

Many people execute this document because they have seen dying inappropriately prolonged in a family member and do not wish this to happen to them. It takes time to think, discuss, get the whole packet together, make copies, and give them to everyone involved, but it is worth it. It has to be done only once, then updated as needed.

Afterword: Geriatrics in a Nutshell

He that would pass the latter part of life with honour and decency must, when he is young, consider that he shall one day be old; and remember when he is old, that he has once been young.
Samuel Johnson, *"The Rambler,"* 1750–1752

What would I like you to remember from this guide?

1. **Aging is living.** We change throughout life. If we are lucky, *we* will join the ranks of the elderly eventually. We will then be more fragile than when younger, with less reserve in body systems, and slower and often incomplete recovery from disease or trauma. Our response to physical stress will be less efficient, and function can be compromised. Our memory, and the ability to learn new skills, although slower in some folks as they age, remain unimpaired with normal aging. Long life and variety of experience enhance many forms of creativity, and the later years are a time when the spirit can

grow and blossom. We *can* choose whether to be a resource or a liability for the next generation.

2. **The longer we live, the more important basic daily functions become.** Loss of function can mean loss of independence, with subsequent infantilization, institutionalization, and poor quality of life. Before every medical intervention, *STOP! THINK!* What will this do to my patient's *function?* If function will be adversely affected, don't proceed unless the benefits are considerable.

3. **More subtle presentation of disease makes diagnosis challenging, but the same path leads to accurate diagnosis at all ages:**

   LISTEN to your patient; he or she is trying to tell you what is wrong.

   LOOK at your patient; observation can give the correct answers.

   TOUCH your patient. There is no substitute for a careful physical examination.

   Order laboratory tests after all this is done with a clear purpose in mind, having weighed the risks and benefits to the patient. (Some diagnostic tests are uncomfortable and not without immediate and longer-term risk.)

   A background of chronic disease with episodes of superimposed acute or subacute disease is usual in many elderly people.

   Physical disease can cause mental changes and vice versa.

4. **Reverse the reversible. Make the irreversible more bearable.** Remember that non-medication treatments such as physical therapy, massage, exercise, meditation, music, and socializing have considerable value.

5. **The elderly are more sensitive to medications.** Be careful and aware when prescribing. Do a risk versus benefit analysis on every item. Remember, "therapeutic" doses can poison the elderly and adversely affect mental and physical function.

6. **The longer we live, the closer we move to death.** The truly excellent practitioner can help the patient and caregivers through this sad time, with finely tuned medical and therapeutic skills, large doses of

compassion, and wise collaboration with the other members of the health team.

Good luck and joy in the practice of our great profession.

MOIRA FORDYCE
SAN FRANCISCO, CALIFORNIA

A

APPENDIX

CAGE Questions

The CAGE questions are used as a screening tool for alcohol overuse.

C **C**ut down—Have you ever felt you ought to cut down on your drinking?

A **A**nger—Have people annoyed you by commenting about your drinking?

G **G**uilt—Have you ever felt bad or guilty about your drinking?

E **E**arly—Have you ever had a drink first thing in the morning to steady your nerves or get rid of a hangover?

A "yes" answer to any of these questions could be significant. Also ask, "How much do you drink each day?" It is important to know how much your patient is drinking daily. Answers such as "A glass of wine" are not precise enough. You need to ask, "How large a glass?"

Alcohol overuse in the elderly is an occult cause of disease, falls, and depression, and every patient should be screened for it and helped to discontinue or moderate this habit.

B

Geriatric Depression Scale (GDS)

Choose the answer that best describes how you felt over the past week.

1. Are you basically satisfied with your life? — Yes/No
2. Have you dropped any of your activities and interests? — Yes/No
3. Do you feel that your life is empty? — Yes/No
4. Do you often get bored? — Yes/No
5. Are you in good spirits most of the time? — Yes/No
6. Are you afraid that something bad is going to happen to you? — Yes/No
7. Do you feel happy most of the time? — Yes/No
8. Do you often feel helpless? — Yes/No
9. Do you prefer to stay at home rather than going out and doing new things? — Yes/No
10. Do you feel that you have more problems with memory than most people? — Yes/No
11. Do you think that it is wonderful to be alive? — Yes/No
12. Do you feel pretty worthless the way you are now? — Yes/No
13. Do you feel full of energy? — Yes/No

14. Do you feel that your situation is
    hopeless?   Yes/No
15. Do you think that most people are
    better off than you are?   Yes/No

This is a good, simple, screening test for geriatric depression. Seven or more inappropriate answers is significant. Five or six inappropriate answers is suggestive of depression.

If the GDS is positive, the patient needs further workup for depression by a geriatrician, or, in some cases, a psychiatrist.

C

Medications Checklist

1. Allergies:

NAME OF MEDICATION   TYPE OF REACTION

_____   _____

_____   _____

_____   _____

_____   _____

2. Please list all the medicines you take that require a doctor's prescription.

_____   _____

_____   _____

_____   _____

_____   _____

_____   _____

3. Please indicate the medicines you take regularly that *do not require* a doctor's prescription (over-the-counter medicines).

	BRAND NAME OF MEDICINE	HOW OFTEN TAKEN? (E.G., DAILY, WEEKLY, MONTHLY)
☐ Antacids	_____	_____
☐ Aspirin	_____	_____
☐ Medicine with aspirin	_____	_____
☐ Arthritis remedies	_____	_____
☐ Calcium supplements	_____	_____
☐ Cold remedies	_____	_____
☐ Cough medicines	_____	_____
☐ Diet pills	_____	_____
☐ Diarrhea preparations	_____	_____
☐ Eye drops	_____	_____
☐ Herbal remedies	_____	_____
☐ Iron or other minerals	_____	_____
☐ Laxatives		
☐ Fiber products/ Metamucil	_____	_____
☐ Motion/travel sickness	_____	_____
☐ Nasal sprays	_____	_____
☐ Pain medicines	_____	_____
☐ Sleep-inducing medication	_____	_____
☐ Tonics	_____	_____
☐ Vitamins	_____	_____
☐ Other	_____	_____

☐ I do not take any over-the-counter medicines.

D

APPENDIX

Evaluation of Skilled Nursing Facility (SNF) Patient

Facility _____ Date _____

Name _____ M/F ___ Age ___ DoB_____

Advance Directives: _____

_____

_____

DPAHC   Yes/No   Contact person _____

Patient informed of diagnosis? Yes/No If no, why

not? _____

_____

_____

Allergies _____ Ht _____ IBW _____ Wt _____

Problem List	Medications

Functional Assessment

ADLs _____ Gait _____ Balance _____

Bowel _____ Bladder _____

Vision _____ Hearing _____

Teeth/mouth _____ Skin _____

Mental Status

3-Item Recall _____ MMS score _____ GDS score _____

Rehabilitation potential _____

_____

Labs _____

_____

SIGNATURE

Name _____ Date _____

Physical Examination and Comments _____

_____

_____

_____

_____

_____

_____

_____

_____

_____

_____

_____

_____

Plan of Treatment _____

_____

_____

_____

_____

_____

_____

_____

_____

SIGNATURE

APPENDIX

Evaluation of the Homebound Patient

Name _____ M/F _____ Age _____ DoB_____

Address _____ Tel # _____

Advance Directives _____

Allergies _____

Problem List	Medications

Comments _____

_____

_____

_____

_____

_____

_____

3-Item Recall _____ MMS score _____ GDS score _____

Rehabilitation potential _____

_____

_____

_____

Labs _____

_____

_____

Plan of Treatment _____

_____

_____

_____

_____

_____

Family Contact _____

_____

SIGNATURE   DATE

F

Mini-Mental State Examination

I carry this with me and use it as an initial screening test of overall intellectual function in my patients. I also use it to monitor changes in mental state at subsequent visits. It remains useful until the patient has significant dementia. When we come to the "Attention and Calculation" section, I ask the patient if he or she is good with numbers. If the patient says no, I either ask him or her to spell "world" backwards or, if the patient cannot read or spell, I ask him or her to do serial 3s instead of serial 7s. If the patient can neither read nor write, I omit the "Close your eyes" command and writing the sentence. In such rare cases, I talk with the patient further about his or her interests and awareness of current events. This gives me a good picture of the patient's overall mental function.

Function	Question or Task	Maximum Score	Score
Orientation	What is the year, season, date, day, month? (5 points) Where are we: state, county, town, hospital, floor? (5 points)	10	

Function	Question or Task	Maximum Score	Score
Registration	Name three objects and ask the patient to repeat the names of the objects (correct response = 1 point). Repeat the names of the three objects until the patient learns them.	3	
Attention and Calculation	Ask the patient to recite serial 7s backward from 100. Stop the patient after five responses (correct response = 1 point). (Or ask the patient to spell WORLD backwards.)	5	
Recall	Ask the patient to repeat the names of the three objects learned above (correct response = 1 point).	3	
Language	Show the patient two common objects (e.g., a pencil and a watch), and ask the patient to identify them (2 points).	2	
	Ask the patient to repeat "no ifs, ands, or buts" (1 point).	1	
	Instruct the patient to follow the three-stage command: "Take a paper in your right hand, fold it in half, and put it on the floor" (3 points).	3	
	Ask the patient to read and obey "Close your eyes" *(below)* (1 point).	1	

Function	Question or Task	Maximum Score	Score
Language	Instruct the patient to write a sentence (1 point). *(Must be a complete sentence. Spelling and grammar don't matter.)*	1	
	Ask the patient to copy a design *(see below)* (1 point).	1	
Total score		30	

Source: Adapted from Folstein MF, Folstein SE, and McHugh PR: "Mini-Mental State," a practical method for grading the cognitive state of patients for the clinician. J Psychiatr Res 12:189–198, 1975.

CLOSE YOUR EYES

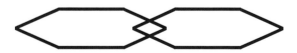

G
APPENDIX

Readings and Resources

TEXTBOOKS

Many excellent textbooks on geriatrics are available. Go to the nearest medical library or bookstore and look through them; then decide which ones will work best for you. The following are my personal favorites, to which I refer often, with my personal comments.

Anderson, F: ***Practical Management of the Elderly,*** ed. 3. Blackwell Scientific Publications, Oxford, 452 pages, 1976. (Distributed in the U.S. by J.B. Lippincott Company, Philadelphia.) ISBN 0-632-0038-4. Hardcover.

This was the first textbook on geriatrics, written by the first professor of geriatrics in the world, a fine man and a superb doctor and teacher. I was privileged to be one of his senior residents back in the 1960s, so I have seen care of the elderly at its very best. I still find this book a fountain of good clinical sense. Sadly, it is out of print, but look for it in second-hand bookshops. It is worth its weight in gold.

Sloan, JP: ***Protocols in Primary Care Geriatrics,*** ed. 2. Springer-Verlag, New York, 206 pages, 1996. ISBN 0-387-94690-X. Paperback.

I like this book. It is short, well written, and to the point, with useful case studies and clinical exercises throughout. Highly recommended for your library.

Hodkinson, HM: *Common Symptoms of Disease in the Elderly,* ed. 2. Blackwell Scientific Publications, Oxford, 147 pages, 1980. ISBN 0-632-00622-6. Paperback.

Brief, but clear and practical, this book is useful for any clinician.

The Merck Manual of Geriatrics, ed. 2. Merck & Co., Rahway, New Jersey, 1200 pages, 1995. ISBN 0-911910-66-2. Hardcover.

I find this a useful, not-too-large reference book.

American Geriatrics Society (DB Reuben et al, eds), *Geriatrics Review Syllabus: A Core Curriculum in Geriatric Medicine,* ed. 3. Kendall/Hunt Publishing, Dubuque, IA, 656 pages, 1998.

The third edition of this large, comprehensive work became available in August 1998. At $285 for American Geriatrics Society (AGS) physician members, $185 for other member categories, and $350 for nonmembers, it might seem expensive, but it is a good self-assessment home-study program, with 200 case-oriented, multiple-choice questions with answers, critiques, and references. In addition, doing the exercises can earn 70 continuing medical education (CME) credits. To order, call Kendall/Hunt Publishing Company at 1-800-228-0810 or fax 1-800-772-9165, or to join AGS and order it, call 1-800-247-4779.

I find that this syllabus works best if a group of health professionals get together at regular intervals and do 10 or so of the questions, discussing them in detail. I consider the syllabus a helpful, useful teaching tool, and, in view of the CME credits, good value for the money. (Check on what attending most courses/symposia/meetings will cost you.)

MEDICAL JOURNALS

I review the *Journal of the American Geriatrics Society* each month and read most of it. Every hospital library has copies of this useful journal. To inquire about it, call the American Geriatrics Society in New York at (212) 308-1414.

I subscribe to ***Journal Watch,*** issued twice each month by the Massachusetts Medical Society, 1440 Main Street, Waltham, MA 02451-1600. It briefly summarizes articles of interest from major medical journals. A year's subscription (24 issues) for U.S. health professionals costs $98 for physicians and $65 for residents, students, nurses, and PAs. To order with a credit card, call 1-800-843-6356 or fax (781) 893-0413.

It is easy to be overwhelmed by the plethora of free medical journals now being thrust upon us, many of them of no great merit. I skim quickly through the contents of these, see who the authors are and where the article or study is from, and sometimes tear out and keep an article, consigning the rest of the journal to the round file.

Reading books and journals is no substitute for seeing patients and talking with your colleagues. Remember, human anatomy does not change. Know it well. Know the basic principles of pathology and apply them to the patients you see. See as many patients as you can. Use your common sense and trust your intuition.

CLINICAL PRACTICE GUIDELINES

The management of chronic pain in older persons. *J Am Geriatr Soc* 46:635–651, 1998.

> This article gives practical guidelines for the management of chronic pain in the elderly. Its main points are covered in this book. They include detailed evaluation of the patient for health, function, and medications; awareness of nonverbal manifestations of pain in the demented patient; elder abuse as a possible contributing factor; long-term pharmacologic management of chronic pain; nonpharmacologic therapies; and referral of patients with intractable pain to other specialties. It concludes with recommendations for health systems that care for older persons.

BOOKS FOR PATIENTS

Over the years I have enjoyed many other excellent books about aging. Here are a few that I have found useful as well as interesting. You can recommend any of the following to your patients:

Comfort, A: *A Good Age.* Simon and Schuster, 224 pages, 1976. ISBN 0-671-24233-4.

> Witty, wise, well written, and full of wonderful advice and beautiful illustrations, this is one of the great classics on aging, now sadly out of print. It was written for a lay audience, but everyone interested in the elderly should read it. Search the second-hand bookstores and library sales.

Berman, PL, and Goldman, C (eds.): *The Ageless Spirit.* Ballantine Books, New York, 283 pages, 1992. ISBN 0-345-36956-4 (Paperback).

> This is a compilation of insightful and inspiring essays on the joys and challenges of growing older from 40 well known senior public figures. You can pick up this book at any time, dive into it for a few minutes, and emerge refreshed.

Morris, V: *How to Care for Aging Parents: A Complete Guide.* Workman Publishing, New York, 460 pages, 1996. ISBN 1-56305-435-3 (Paperback).

> This well-written, well-presented book for a lay audience is full of useful information. Health professionals who work with the elderly can learn a lot from reading this.

Whiting Little, D: *Home Care for the Dying.* The Dial Press, Doubleday & Company, Inc., Garden City NY, 316 pages, 1985. ISBN 0-385-27750-4 (Paperback).

> This is an excellent book, full of practical advice, good sense and compassion. The author is nonmedical and wrote this book after caring at home for her beloved grandmother for 6 months before she died. Well worth reading at least once. Sadly, it is now out of print.

RESOURCES

Following is a list of some helpful resources for patients and their families. More detailed lists can usually be obtained from the medical social work department at your local hospital, most senior citizen centers, and the local area Agency on Aging.

ABA Commission on Legal Problems of the Elderly
American Bar Association, 740 Fifteenth St., NW, Washington DC 20005-1022
(202) 662-8690, Fax (202) 662-8698
Web site:
http://www.abanet.org/elderly/home.html

This commission offers information and links to other web sites relating to Social Security, advance directives, and many other topics with legal implications.

Alzheimer's Association
919 North Michigan Avenue, Suite 1000, Chicago, IL 60611-1626
1-800-272-3900. Web site **http://www.alz.org**

This association offers information and advice for patients with Alzheimer's dementia and their families. A list of local chapters is available.

American Association of Retired Persons
601 E Street, NW, Washington, DC 20049
(202) 434-2277. Web site **http://www.aarp.org**

AARP is a nonprofit, nonpartisan organization with more than 32 million members aged 50 and over. Not all members are retired, in spite of the title. The association's aims are to improve the lives of older Americans through service, advocacy, education, and volunteer efforts. Its political muscle is large and growing larger. It is an excellent resource for every aspect of aging—medical, social, and financial.

American Diabetes Association
1660 Duke Street, Alexandria, VA 22314
1-800-232-3472. Web site **http://www.diabetes.org**

Information, leaflets, and other materials are available for people with diabetes.

American Parkinson Disease Association

1250 Hylan Blvd, Suite 4B, Staten Island, NY 10305-1946
1-800-223-2732.
Web site **http://www.apdaparkinson.com**

The number shown is a hotline for information about Parkinson's disease.

Cancer Information Service

National Cancer Institute, Bldg 31, Room 10A 24, Bethesda, MD 20892
1-800-422-6237

The number shown is a hotline for cancer patients and their families.

Eldercare Locator

Department of Health and Human Services
1-800-677-1116

This locator helps to identify local resources for the elderly.

Health Care Financing Administration

Mailstop C2-25-11, 7500 Security Blvd, Baltimore, MD 21244
1-800-638-6833

This is the Medicare hotline.

National Association for Home Care

519 C St, NE, Washington, DC 20002
(202) 547-7424. Web site **http://www.nahc.org**

Information about federally funded home care programs is provided.

National Hospice Organization

1901 North Moore St., Suite 901, Arlington VA 22209
(703) 243-5900

This organization has resources related to death and dying (including the death of pets) and the hospice movement.

National Institute on Aging Information Center
P.O. Box 8057, Gaithersburg, MD 20898-8057
1-800-222-2225. Web site **http://www.nih.gov/nia**

Information is available on a wide range of aging-related topics.

National Rehabilitation Information Center
8455 Colesville Rd, Suite 935, Silver Spring, MD 20910-3319
1-800-346-2742.
Web site **http://www.cais.net/naric**

Information about rehabilitation, physical therapy, and occupational therapy is available.

National Stroke Association
8480 East Orchard Rd, Suite 1000, Englewood, CO 80111-5015
(303) 649-9299. Web site **http://www.stroke.org**

This association provides information for stroke patients and their families.

Where to Find More Resources

The following are two useful, comprehensive publications about resources:

Physician's National Resource Directory. MultiMedia HealthCare/Freedom, LLC, Office Center at Princeton Meadows, Bldg 300, Plainsborough NJ 08536. Phone (609) 275-3800, Fax (609) 275-4779.

Cheney, WJ, et al: *The Second 50 Years: A Reference Manual for Senior Citizens.* Writers Consortium, 5443 Stag Mountain Rd., Weed CA 96094. 1-800-887-5526. Web site: **http://seniors-site.com**

This web site not only is a source for obtaining the book, but also includes information on other resources for seniors.

H
APPENDIX

Acronyms and Mnemonics

Acronym or Mnemonic	Meaning	Where to Look for Explanation
AID	Risk factors for poor nutrition in the elderly	Chapter 18, p. 163
BOB	Beware of bleeding!	Chapters 6 and 7, pp. 47, 50, 53
CAGE	Screening for alcohol overuse	Appendix A, p. 218
CARE	Principles of prescribing for the elderly	Chapter 16, p. 146
DEEM	Management of the diabetic	Chapter 18, p. 163
DEMENTIA	Potentially treatable causes of confusion in the elderly	Chapter 9, pp. 85–86
DIPS	Risk factors for pressure sores	Chapter 8, p. 64
DRIP	Causes of transient incontinence	Chapter 8, p. 67
ICM (I See 'Em)	Causes of delirium	Chapter 9, p. 83

I

Abbreviations

AARP. American Association of Retired Persons
AD. Alzheimer's dementia
ADLs. Activities of daily living
AF. Atrial fibrillation
ALS. Amyotrophic lateral sclerosis
APTT. Activated partial thromboplastin time
ASA. Acetylsalicylic acid (aspirin)
ASCVD. Arteriosclerotic cardiovascular disease
BID. Twice daily
BOB. Beware of bleeding
BP. Blood pressure
BPH. Benign prostatic hypertrophy
BUN. Blood urea nitrogen
CAD. Coronary artery disease
CBC. Complete blood count
CHF. Congestive heart failure
COPD. Chronic obstructive pulmonary disease
CPR. Cardiopulmonary resuscitation
CVA. Cerebrovascular accident
DJD. Degenerative joint disease
DM. Diabetes mellitus
DPAHC. Durable power of attorney for health care
DVT. Deep vein thrombosis
ECG. Electrocardiogram
ECT. Electroconvulsive therapy
EEG. Electroencephalogram
GI(T). Gastrointestinal (tract)
GT. Gastrostomy tube

GU. Genitourinary
Hb, Hgb. Hemoglobin
HRT. Hormone replacement therapy
HS. At bedtime
HTN. Hypertension
IADLs. Instrumental activities of daily living
IBW. Ideal body weight
IDDM. Insulin-dependent diabetes mellitus
IHD. Ischemic heart disease
IM. Intramuscular(ly)
INR. International normalized ratio
IU. International units
IV. Intravenous(ly)
KISS. Keep it simple, sweetie
LVH. Left ventricular hypertrophy
MAOI. Monoamine oxidase inhibitor
MCV. Mean corpuscular volume
MI. Myocardial infarction
MS. Morphine sulfate (also Multiple Sclerosis)
NG. Nasogastric
NIDDM. Non-insulin-dependent diabetes mellitus
NSAID. Nonsteroidal anti-inflammatory drug
OT. Occupational therapy (or therapist)
PA. Pernicious anemia (also Physician assistant)
PE. Pulmonary embolism (also Physical Examination)
po. By mouth, orally
prn. As needed
PT. Prothrombin time (also Physical therapy)
PVD. Peripheral vascular disease
PVS. Persistent vegetative state
Q. Every, as in "Q 4h"
QD. Daily
QID. Four times daily
QOD. Every other day
SC. Subcutaneous(ly)
SL. Sublingual(ly)
SNF. Skilled nursing facility ("nursing home")
SSRI. Selective serotonin reuptake inhibitor
STD. Sexually transmitted disease
TB. Tuberculosis
TENS. Transcutaneous nerve stimulation
TGF. Transforming growth factor
TIA. Transient ischemic attack

TID. Three times daily
TSH. Thyroid stimulating hormone (thyrotropin)
UA. Urinalysis
URI. Upper respiratory infection
UTI. Urinary tract infection
VA. Veterans Administration
WBC. White blood count (or cell)

Index

An "f" following a page number indicates a figure;
a "t" indicates a table.